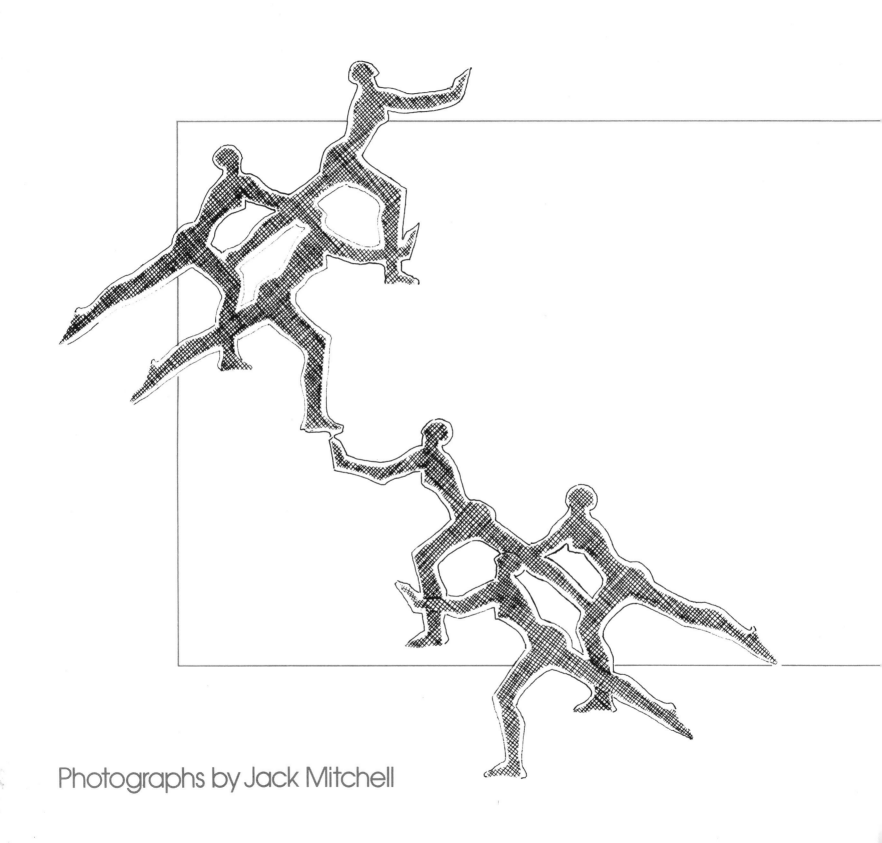

Photographs by Jack Mitchell

the articulate body

sidi hessel

Designed and Illustrated by the author

St. Martin's Press New York

Copyright© 1978 by Sidi Hessel
All rights reserved. For information, write:
St. Martin's Press
175 Fifth Avenue
New York, N.Y. 10010
Manufactured in the United States of America
Library of Congress Catalog Card Number: 77-9180
Library of Congress Cataloging in Publication Data
Hessel, Sidi.
    The articulate body.
    1.   Exercise for women.   2.   Joints—Range of
motion.   3.   Posture.   I.   Title.
RA781.H476   613.7'045   77-9180
ISBN 0-312-05483-1

for Sandra D. McCormack

In the course of writing this book I received a great deal of help. I thank my editors Thomas J. McCormack and Patricia McNees Mancini for their invaluable criticism and guidance and my husband Bernard Hans Hessel for his unfailing patience and support.

I am indebted to my dear friend Winnie Schaeffer for many excellent suggestions as well as the timing and testing of all the programs and to Tim McGuire, Sally Richardson and Joanne Michaels for helping to smooth the way. Thanks are also due to Carol Robson for assisting with design decisions and to Tony Gerber for meticulously copy-editing the manuscript.

My heartfelt thanks and appreciation for their kind attentions and encouragement go to Rose and Julius Schwartz, Caroline Newhouse (Mrs. Theo Newhouse), Shirley Mandel (Mrs. Jack Mandel), Carolyn Ambuter (Mrs. Joseph Ambuter), Dorshka and Samson Raphaelson, Phillip Winter and to my dear students—past and present.

Contents

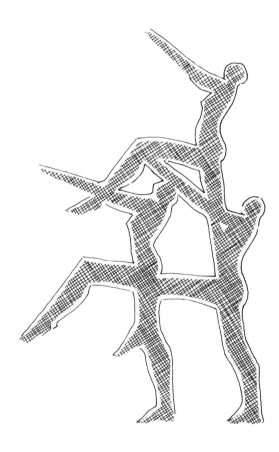

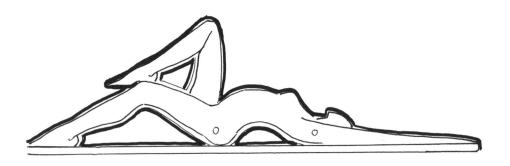

the point of articulation

This book is about how you look, how you feel, and how you move. It will restore and enhance your body's appearance, sensations, and performance—but in case this suggests a concern solely with physical beauty and fitness, I should say at once that the benefits extend equally to the mind and spirit. Body and mind are in effect inseparable. I don't mean anything mystical by this. This is not a book of ineffable mystiques, but of physical techniques. There will be no talk about mind control, alpha waves, or the like. Instead, there will be a number of special physical movements and adjustments carried out in precise ways.

And you can count on this: the techniques of physical training described here will rejuvenate and revitalize your mind and spirit more assuredly than the very newest 5,000-year-old method from the Orient.

When I say body and mind are inseparable, I mean this: when our bodies lose shape, when tension, stiffness, or pain nag at us constantly, when our energy is sapped by dysfunctions we associate with "age," when we sense the slipping away of our ability to move with grace, dispatch, or pleasure, when we seem to lose touch with our bodies—the impact on our spirit is direct and undeniable. All these physical woes and more are what the program in this book will reverse.

Other popular systems purporting to enhance body and spirit have their benefits, but within an elaborate system the specific element that works is often unrecognized, buried beneath an irrelevant ritual, like a speck of vitamin in a pound of food. My system focuses steadily on the key pragmatic physical factors that determine how your body feels, looks, and moves. I believe these are the factors that in truth underlie much of what is beneficial in such disparate systems as T'ai Chi Ch'uan and bioenergetics, yoga and sports training, dance and sleep-position therapy.

Your training will focus solely on the beneficial elements, avoiding the irrelevant and harmful, and your techniques will be geared to what you can accomplish naturally. When I ask you to move in certain precise ways, you'll be able to do so. Your body is under your direct control and you won't be asked to do a movement before you are prepared to do it correctly. Be assured that learning to move correctly will reward you both physically and psychologically.

With all the dire connotations "physical training" brings to mind, I want to say at once that this training will be unlike any other. Perhaps the best way to convey what it's like is to say what it is not, to contrast it with more familiar techniques.

For one thing, it is not "exercise." It involves no fierce and violent motion, no heavy breathing, no rapid, strenuous exertions—not because it is an easy system that requires no effort, but because those things actually work against the goals we want to achieve.

What we aim to develop is suppleness and resilience, mobility and agility, body sensitivity, balanced posture, the tone and shape that characterize a body's natural comeliness. Forced limbering techniques have simply proved to be ineffective at achieving any of these. We shall also want to develop power and endurance, but only to the extent needed to move with the pleasure, grace, and efficiency of normal youthfulness. This is not the book for people who want to run a 4-minute mile or to lift 500 pounds. I am concerned with extending the range of your normal activity so that you can function at a high energy level all day without collapsing with fatigue.

More particularly, the usual exercise program tends to emphasize muscle contraction; this program emphasizes muscle elongation. I will use the word "stretching" a good deal, but again, I won't be asking for arduous efforts.

Other programs focus on developing large, obvious muscles. This program, while not ignoring the larger muscles, will regularly focus on smaller muscles and on tendons and joints, often reawakening muscles you were not even aware you had. I've seldom met a woman intensely concerned about her biceps, but the inner surfaces of the upper arms concern many of us. "Why do they appear so flabby? Why are they losing their shape?" Because their tone and shape depend on the regular stimulation of certain small muscle groups that go virtually uncalled-upon throughout adult life. Reacquaint yourself with these muscles to make them respond. For many, I guarantee, it will be like meeting a long-lost friend. It may seem like a game, but reestablishing and maintaining contact with all parts of your body is immensely important.

Another reason we'll concentrate on smaller muscle groups is that very often smaller muscles are the cause of trouble their larger neighbors are blamed for. Stiffness in the knee joint, for example, is usually caused by a loss of flexibility in several small, obscure, and deeply imbedded muscles surrounding the joint. When these are inflexible, they bind the knee like a series of tapes and bandages. Stretching the larger muscles of the calves and thighs will not touch the real problem.

Many training programs involve rapid, quickly repeated actions, and stress maximum effort. In this system, the key is minimum effort, mainly because maximum effort will not produce the desired results. If you strain at what I describe, you'll be doing the movement wrong. You'll be asked to move slowly and to relax after each effort, not to make things easy for you, but to prevent fatigue, by insuring a balanced flow of oxygen to the muscles and the removal of energy waste products from the muscles. Fatigue ultimately inhibits movement, and inhibition of movement is exactly what we're fighting.

The relaxation we ask for between movements is of a special kind: it is a total release that is essential to inducing the flexibility and resilience that muscles and tendons should have. Some of your muscles may be too short, always semi-contracted and tense even during "relaxation." Others may be too long, lacking tone and shape and allowing for hyperextensions which are havoc on joints. One aim of this training is to stimulate muscles to revert to their natural length when at rest, eliminating both tension and slackness, improving the shape of the body, and giving muscles the right tone for perfect responsiveness.

Another way in which this training will differ from other programs concerns your current limits of comfortable movement. The aim here will be not to urge you to exceed them, but to extend them. And extend them you will, without pain. Agony is out, not only because the natural impulse is to avoid it—and thus to avoid the training that causes it—but also because it creates fatigue and induces precisely the tensions we're trying to expel.

The goals we want to achieve—suppleness, agility, revitalized body sensitivity, the rejuvenation of shape and tone, a buoyant step, a pleasure and command in all our bodily motions, along with the totally vibrant and attractive projection of our selves that these things insure—all of these goals will proceed from certain basic dynamic faculties that this program will develop to their full potential.

One of these faculties is mobility—the free and full action that every joint, tendon, and muscle in your body is capable of. Before long-forgotten muscles will respond, you need to develop the minimum mobility to connect with those muscles. Articulations, the section designed to increase mobility, comes first because that first connection is likely to be less than perfect.

Another faculty is muscle sense, body awareness, the control and consciousness of their physical being that great athletes and dancers enjoy. You will frequently encounter the word "feel" in this book. Feeling, and remembering what you have felt, are essential to developing kinesthesia, your muscle sense. You will be asked to perform a certain movement and to notice the sensation it produces. For every action, no matter how small, there is a reaction to be felt. You're bound to notice the strong sensations—in your calf when you arch your foot, for example, or in your shoulder when you lift your arm—but you'll be asked to concentrate on small, less obvious, but absolutely crucial muscles as they contract, elongate, or relax. Once you have learned to identify motions with sensations, you can memorize, direct, and summon the feelings at will. You can develop the ability to get in touch with your body and to "see" yourself in the round, gaining a total sense of the position, size, weight, and motion of every part of your body. It is an exhilarating feeling, one that will make you look vibrantly alive and responsive, attributes that will heighten your capacity for pleasure—from your sexuality to your tennis game. A strong, glorious kinesthetic sense is the very fabric of self-awareness.

Although muscle sense is a natural faculty, it can atrophy as surely as a muscle itself. To cultivate this faculty, I will be asking for your attention. I will ask you to feel your responses the way a music appreciation teacher might ask you to listen for the oboes in an orchestra; it will take concentration but you'll soon be rewarded by registering the whole magnificent orchestration of your body.

The dynamic faculties your training will next develop are power and control. You need both in order to maintain what may also be called a faculty—good posture. But you can't acquire the kind of power and control you need unless you strengthen weak and neglected muscle groups and learn to activate your existing, though often dormant, support muscles.

In the section on posture, I will explain that the poor alignment responsible for poor posture is almost always caused by a failure to use your antigravity equipment efficiently.

Mobility, muscle sense, power, and control—with these faculties functioning at their full potential, we're ready to combat the enemies of the articulate body. Slack muscles will be toned. Stiffness and tensions will be banished. So will muscle weakness, poor posture, bad circulation, and insufficient oxygen intake. And so shall nerve fatigue, blocked sensation, muscle binding, and muscle locking.

At the heart of much of what we'll be doing is stretching. <u>Stretching</u> will make your body limber, supple, and flexible—and therefore healthier, shapelier, more efficient and pleasurable in motion, stronger and more adroit. More and more athletes and performers have made stretching part of their daily practice.

More important to many of us, stretching is a natural tranquilizer, making our bodies more efficient at rest. Simply sitting or standing upright is an onerous task for many. And consider sleep: many people, as they live with unnecessary muscle and tendon rigidity, find that they sleep in fewer and fewer positions. Somehow their sleep is less satisfying. They get out of bed aching rather than refreshed. Seeing the wonderful sprawl of a sleeping child, they say, "How I wish I could still do that!" But they can! And you can too.

Much attention in this book will be paid to the joints, which are pivotal to much of what we want to accomplish. Why call the book <u>"The Articulate Body"</u>? I wanted the title to summon up the basic meaning of <u>articulate</u>, having to do with being jointed, or having joints. A great deal of our focus throughout will be on where the joints are, how they work, and how to restore their full mobility. I say "where they are" because, surprisingly, many of us don't know the exact location of our joints. For example, when you stand erect and bend over to touch your toes, chances are you'll do it as though your torso were joined to your legs somewhere around your lower back. Actually, your torso joins your legs at the hip joints. And the hip joints are not at the "crests of the pelvis," those two bony prominences about navel-high, but are located where the long thighbones join the pelvic girdle—which is much lower and in toward the groin. What difference does it make? Just this: if you bend from the lower back and not from the hip joints, you are putting undue strain on your spine and lower back muscles. You will damage them, causing yourself pain and needless exertion. You'll only reach your toes after lots of work. And when you do you will have bypassed the muscles that need toning—bending from the lower back does nothing for the buttocks or thighs.

In my initial classes I often ask women to bend over and touch their toes. Regularly, they bend from the lower back and they usually don't get within 5 inches of the floor. When I show them how to bend from the hip joints, they are often astonished to find themselves touching the ground with all ten fingers. They do this without strain or pain, while toning and shaping exactly the areas they're interested in.

Do you know how many joints there are in the foot and ankle alone? Probably not, because you regularly move so few of them. When the muscles and tendons around these joints are properly activated through gentle stretches and releases, the effect is marvelous. Not only do ankle and foot articulations relieve over-all tensions, they also help to reshape the entire ankle area. Women whose ankles tend to accumulate fluid can perceive the disappearance of puffiness as joint articulation dissipates excess fluid in a kind of milking action.

The point where bone joins with bone is the point of articulation, and what we want to develop is full, free, comfortable articulation. If you were to gain nothing else from this book, that alone could change your whole sense of your body and your self. And this touches on the other sense of "articulate" that I want to conjure up: the sense of skillful, fluent self-expression. The articulate body expresses and projects the vitality of its owner. It is not too much to say that you in your normal life can possess and project exactly the radiant aura of body awareness, control, and vibrancy that makes a young dancer so exciting.

The parallel with a young dancer is particularly apt for the teenagers and young actresses who come to my studio, but let me make it clear that this program has no age limits. Some of my students are in their sixties, and they do not believe that maturity is sufficient reason for their bodies to let them down. Mobility should last a lifetime and so should a conscious sense of well-being—not just the absence of pain, fatigue, or discomfort, but a positive sense of feeling good that allows you to function on all cylinders and enjoy life.

Too many of us resign ourselves to a steady depletion of energy and the gradual impoverishment of our bodies; we live at only a fraction of our capacity, functioning below par because we haven't the slightest inkling of the body's potential. If you feel that locked within you is a self crying out for physical expression but rendered mute and inglorious by a body that was once a home and is now a prison—if your body longs to regain the sublime vocabulary of youth—then I think The Articulate Body is the book for you.

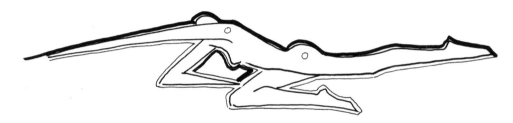

about your program

In forty years of teaching I have never discovered a formula for instant perfection. Experience has also taught me that bodies can be improved without strenuous exertion. Your program is therefore neither a crash course nor a regimen of exhausting exercise, but rather a progressive training plan based on three easy-to-learn techniques that will help to develop your body's full potential—albeit gradually.

How long this will take depends on your condition as you begin, and on whether you practice regularly. To make daily practice stimulating, your program features a revolving lesson plan, in which new movements are added regularly. To relieve you of guesswork, there are four programs to guide you toward lasting results. Don't consider the early and often dramatic changes you will see in yourself as your final achievement. The loss of a few inches here and there is only a small part of what your training will eventually yield.

Although I designed this program for women, it can be shared with all members of your family. Part 1, Articulations, is devoted to relaxation and mobility training. Dispelling tensions and freeing the joints of the body are as beneficial to men as to women. And because the movements in this section demand little energy, all the members of your family will find them helpful.

In Part 2, Posture, the focus is on body awareness, correct alignment, and good posture. Since it is important to establish good postural habits early in life, the second part of this section—Posture Toning—will be useful for young children and teenagers of both sexes.

A special technique in Part 3, The Book of Stretches, will help to tone and shape your body and improve your mobility and coordination. Moving easily and well is essential to everyone's well-being, and the results of this training—coordination and flexibility, linked to strength—are as valuable to a football player as to a woman walking down the street.

To get the most out of this program, follow its basic order and practice regularly at least 20 or, ideally, 30 minutes a day. If you are too busy to practice on schedule, or if you have to travel, use the mini-program on page 133. Don't wear anything binding, and practice in a well-ventilated room—without interruption if possible. Use a soft mat, a rug, or a large bath towel for your floor work; do seated work on a straight-backed chair with a firm seat.

Handling a book as you move can be a problem so either read ahead and memorize your instructions, or use a typing stand or cookbook holder. We have tested both with success.

Articulations

the ABC of body language

Articulation—or movement of your joints—is the ABC of body language. In this first, important part of your training, you will explore and develop the full range of motion in your joints.

Although nothing contributes as much to your sense of well-being as the ability to move with a minimum expenditure of energy, movement is usually identified with effort. And it is true that certain kinds of activity require effort, but during Articulations you will accomplish more when you control your energy output.

Healthy joints, like fine mechanical devices, operate without friction. When a delicate precision instrument fails to function with ease, skilled mechanics never use force—instead, they apply a lubricant and allow time for it to penetrate between the unyielding parts.

This is precisely the attitude you should adopt toward the joints of your body. Resist making efforts that are out of proportion to actual needs. Don't <u>strive</u> to move; <u>allow</u> yourself to move. If you encounter any resistance, don't blame it on your joints. Joint "stiffness," common even in young women, is normally due not to dysfunction of the joints but to tensions in the muscles that surround them.

Intense, exaggerated efforts cannot free your joints. The only reliable remedy for tensions that inhibit your mobility is a special kind of relaxation, which you induce with a series of small, almost effortless, but sensitively executed movements—<u>Articulations.</u>

Try rotating your wrist as if you were scooping a heavy mass of clay out of a bowl. Then, controlling your energy output, repeat the movement and pretend that you are gathering up a handful of whipped cream.

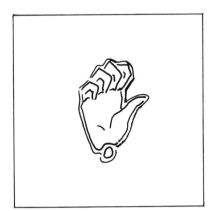

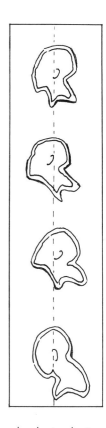

Cultivating this quality of relaxed movement will make you aware of yourself in a new way and will allow your joints to operate smoothly and effortlessly, like parts of a well-oiled machine. This is the secret behind the loose-limbed grace of athletes, dancers, and jungle cats.

The value of Articulations that activate small, and often neglected, muscle groups cannot be overestimated. Recent research by medical experts has shown that osteoporosis—the bone loss that may contribute to the fractures suffered by older people—is found four times more frequently in women than men, and that normal women after the age of 35 have a bone loss of 10 percent a decade.

Dr. Louis V. Avioli, Professor of Medicine at the Washington University School of Medicine in St. Louis, has stated, "Muscle mass seems very important to the integrity of bone, and the day-by-day muscles pulling through tendons insertions stimulates formation of bone."

Unless you are relaxed enough for your joints to move freely, you cannot pull or stretch your tendons and muscles fully. A basic understanding of your body structure and the role of the joints in your body's movement will help you to relax.

Your body is designed along a central, upright axis. Your skull, rib cage, spine, and pelvis enclose and protect your vital organs. The bones of your limbs, like levers united by joints, move your body. Your joints are held in place by somewhat elastic, tough, bandlike ligaments. Your bones serve as the attachment for strong wirelike tendons, which anchor your muscles to your frame. Muscles of various shapes and size wind in many layers like straps and harnesses around your skeletal structure, giving your body support, volume, and shape.

The shapes of your joints—bows, angles, blades, cages, rings, sockets, and spheres—determine their function and degree of mobility.

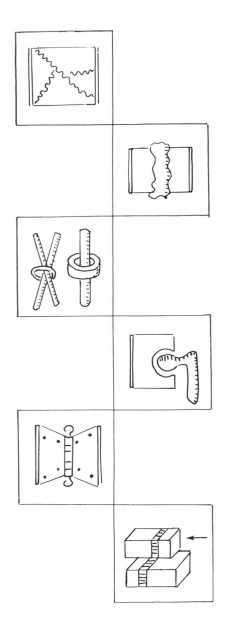

The sawtooth-edged seams of your skull are immovable after infancy.

The joints that unite the segments of your spinal column, and those that unite your ribs to your breastbone, have only passive movement (they respond to the movement of your body by yielding, and allow your rib cage to expand).

The joint at the base of your skull pivots, and those in your forearms and lower legs swivel.

The ball-and-socket joints of your shoulders and hips rotate with great freedom.

The hinge joints of your elbows, knees, fingers and toes have angular, one-directional movement.

The joints of your wrists and ankles glide plane to plane, united by retaining ligaments.

Joints are capable of different kinds of movement. For example, the knuckles are hinge joints, yet each finger is also capable of slight rotation.

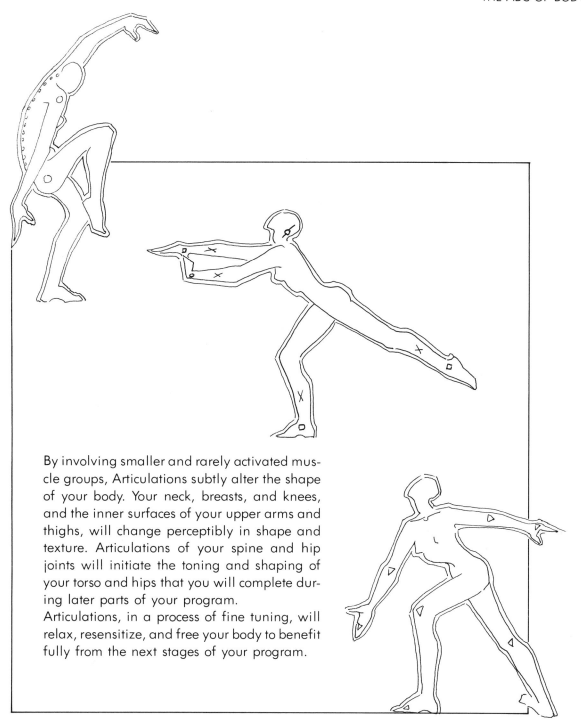

By involving smaller and rarely activated muscle groups, Articulations subtly alter the shape of your body. Your neck, breasts, and knees, and the inner surfaces of your upper arms and thighs, will change perceptibly in shape and texture. Articulations of your spine and hip joints will initiate the toning and shaping of your torso and hips that you will complete during later parts of your program.

Articulations, in a process of fine tuning, will relax, resensitize, and free your body to benefit fully from the next stages of your program.

Articulations From Head to Toe

During your initial training, you will gain access to your body's resources by developing the full range of motion in your joints. Since relaxation is indispensable to total mobility, this part of your training will not make great demands on your energy; instead, it will call for concentration and control.

To get a full grasp of how your body operates, move slowly and never force your joints beyond their present capacity. Remember that during Articulations you accomplish far more by doing less.

Articulations are practiced in the following order:

Set A   The Jaws, Neck and Shoulders
Set B   The Shoulder Joints and Elbows
Set C   The Wrists and Fingers
Set D   The Spine
Set E   The Hips and Knees
Set F   The Ankles and Toes

program

"Once each" may mean once each, or once on each side, or once in each direction, whichever applies.

1)   Practice for 1 day:

Set A movements, all repeats.

2)   Practice for 1 day:

Set A movements, once each.

Set B movements, all repeats.

3)   Practice for 1 day:

Set A, Set B movements, once each.

Set C movements, all repeats.

4)   Practice for 1 day:

Set A, Set B, Set C movements, once each.

Set D movements, all repeats.

5)   Practice for 1 day:

Set A, Set B, Set C, Set D movements, once each.

Set E movements, all repeats.

6)   Practice for 1 day:

Set A, Set B, Set C, Set D, Set E movements, once each.

Set F movements, all repeats.

After you have completed all of the sets, Articulations will continue to be an important part of your daily practice.

the jaws

Jaws are often compressed and tense. One-sided chewing causes an imbalance of facial muscle tone, as well as strain that may result in a tendency to grind the teeth at night. To relax the jaws, before retiring repeat the first two Articulations 8 times each in addition to your daily practice.

yawning

Sit well back in a straight-backed chair, feet slightly apart, hands in your lap. Let your jaw drop. With your mouth open, rest the tip of your tongue lightly against the inner surface of your lower front teeth. With tongue in place, slowly open your mouth wide as if to yawn. Hold for a slow count of 3. Close your mouth. Relax.

Do this 3 times.

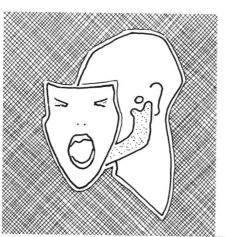

sliding

Sit as before. Lift your chin slightly and let your jaw drop. With your mouth open, rest the tip of your tongue lightly against the inner surface of your upper front teeth. With tongue in place, slide your lower jaw forward, then slide it slowly and smoothly from side to side. Close your mouth. Relax.

Do this 6 times.

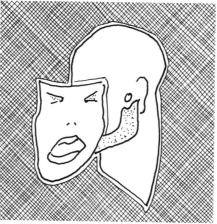

the atlas

Where the base of the skull meets the top of the neck is a unique joint, composed of the two highest vertebrae of the neck. The first segment, called the atlas after the Greek giant of legend who bore up the heavens, is a bony ring attached to the skull. Directly beneath it is the second segment, the axis, which has a toothlike projection that rises from its center and penetrates the ring. This joint is a pivot, permitting great freedom of motion in turning, tilting, nodding, lifting, and rotating the head.

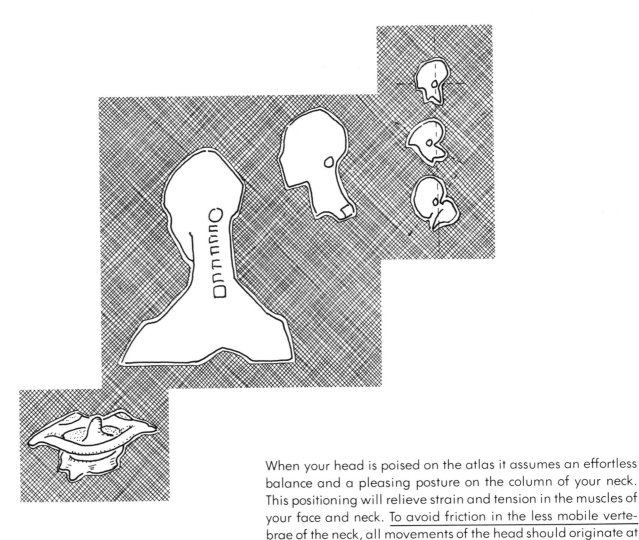

When your head is poised on the atlas it assumes an effortless balance and a pleasing posture on the column of your neck. This positioning will relieve strain and tension in the muscles of your face and neck. To avoid friction in the less mobile vertebrae of the neck, all movements of the head should originate at the atlas.
Place your index finger on the most prominent vertebra at the base of your neck. Probe upward along the neck with your finger until you feel a small hollow near the base of your skull. This is the location of your atlas.

the neck

Painful neck tension is a familiar symptom. If you suffer from neck tension, practice Set A movements as often as instructed for several days, and also before bedtime.

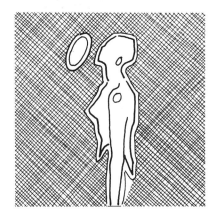

circling

Sit upright, hands in your lap. Plan to keep your neck still. Pretend that you are holding a round hand mirror close to your face. Describe its circumference with the tip of your nose. Move slowly clockwise, then counterclockwise. Feel your neck muscles relaxing.

Do this 3 times in each direction.

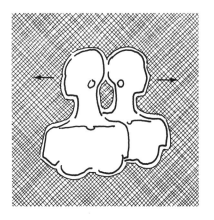

turning

Sit as before. Without tilting your face, turn your head slowly to the right until you feel the first resistance. Relax and stretch your neck, then continue to turn right as far as comfort will allow. Slowly move your head back to center. Relax.

Do this 3 times in each direction.

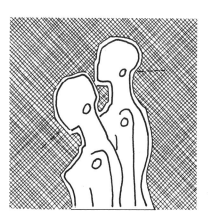

nodding

Sit as before. Keeping your neck straight and still, slowly lower your chin no more than an inch. Hold for a slow count of 3. Moving from the atlas return to the starting position. Feel the muscles of your forehead and the back of your scalp relaxing.

Do this 6 times.

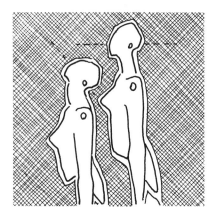

tilting back

Sit upright, feet slightly apart, arms relaxed at your sides. Keeping your back straight, slowly lift your chin until the back of your head rests lightly against the lowest part of the back of your neck; open your mouth slightly. Move slowly upward from the back of the neck until your head is poised on the atlas. Feel a sense of ease and weightlessness.

Do this 4 times.

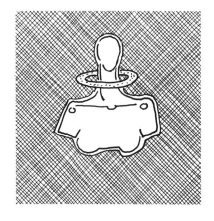

high rotations

Sit as before. Lift your chin and, combining the motions of nodding, tilting, and turning, slowly roll your head high at the atlas. Think of the atlas as a ball-bearing joint, and roll your head in a full circle without straining or pressing. You may hear a slight crackling sound, which is harmless.

Do this 3 times in each direction.

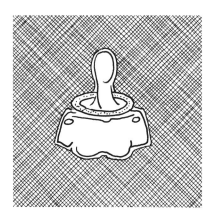

low rotations

Read this before starting. Sit tall, arms relaxed at your sides. Lift your shoulders and plan to keep them high. Open your mouth and lift your chin until the back of your head is lightly cushioned on your shoulders. Roll your head slowly toward your right shoulder. Starting with your chin against your right collarbone, roll your head toward your left shoulder, then up and over your left shoulder and back to center. Lower your shoulders. Relax.

Do this 3 times in each direction.

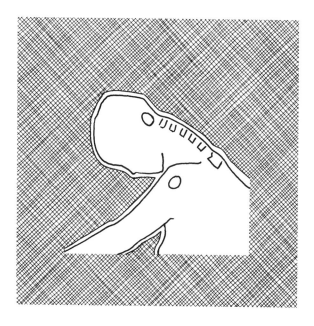

curved rotations

When your neck is upright, the bony segments at its back are close together. When you stretch your neck by moving your head forward and down, these segments separate slightly.

Sit upright with hands on your knees. Slowly lower your chin to your chest. Allow your back to curve. Feel your neck relaxing and stretching. Without forcing, move your chin slowly from side to side. Raise your head and resume starting position.

Do this 6 times.

the shoulders

Your collarbones, breastbone, and shoulder blades interact to form your shoulder girdle. Tensions often accumulate between your shoulder blades and at the crest of your shoulders. Two movements are especially helpful in relieving these tensions: (a) arching and (b) curving.

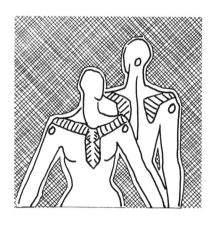

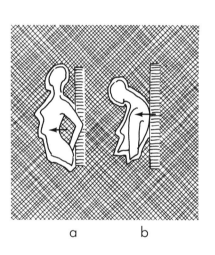

a   b

the collarbones

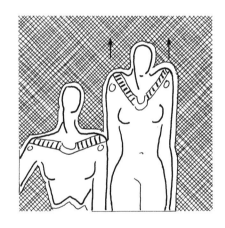

lifting

Sit upright, arms relaxed at your sides. Do not bend your arms or move your shoulders back. Starting from the outer ends of your collarbones, raise your shoulders toward your ears. Slowly lower your shoulders and lengthen your neck without lifting your chin. Relax.

Do this 4 times.

the shoulder blades

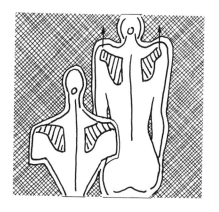

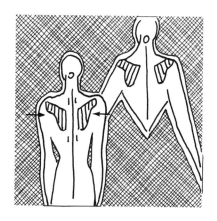

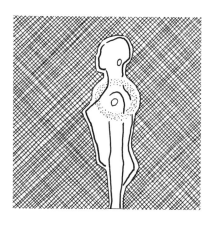

shoulder rotations

Sit upright, feet slightly apart. Plan to keep your arms straight and relaxed at your sides. With neck relaxed, and in one slow, continuous motion, move your shoulders slightly forward. Then raise them as high as possible without pressing. Then roll them back and down, allowing your chest to lift. Relax. Rotate first from front to back, then from back to front.

Do this 3 times in each direction.

lifting

Sit upright, hands in your lap. Move your shoulders slightly forward without lifting them. Lower your head and allow your spine to curve as you move your shoulder blades upward as far as possible. Feel your upper back curving and stretching. Lower your shoulders and resume your starting position.

Do this 3 times.

compressing

Sit upright, arms straight along your sides, palms facing front. Lift your chin slightly and gently arch your back. Raise your shoulders high, then press them back firmly. Feel a strong compression in the center of your upper back. Press your elbows back and down to increase the compression. Relax.

Do this 4 times.

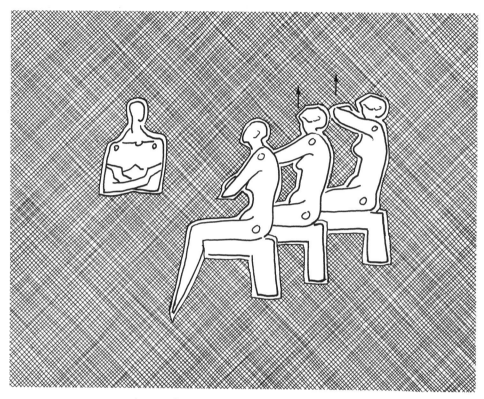

separating the shoulder blades

Read this before starting.

Sit with legs wide apart. Cross your arms and slump. Plan to remain in this position. Lift your shoulders, then press them forward slightly. Feel the distance between your shoulder blades increasing. Press the base of your neck back. Feel a pressure at the back of the neck. Relax in position. Roll your head back until it rests on your shoulders and open your mouth. Slowly raise your elbows, pressing them forward until they are slightly above shoulder level. Lower your arms and resume the starting position.

Do this 3 times.

the shoulder joints

Shoulder joints have the greatest range of movement in your body. For greater freedom of movement, <u>always lift your rib cage slightly before raising your arms above shoulder level.</u>

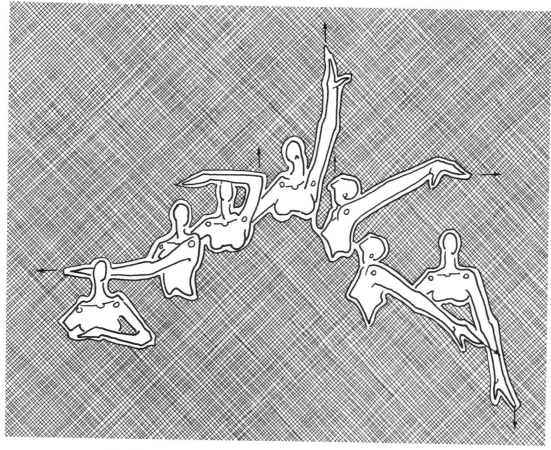

arm rotations

Stand upright, feet slightly apart and turned out, arms relaxed. Shift your weight to the balls of your feet. Place your left hand, palm down, against the center of your chest.

Without allowing your shoulder to follow, move your left arm toward the right until it is almost straight.

Lift your rib cage, then bend and lift your left elbow until your forearm is just above your head.

With your left thumb pointing back, straighten your arm. Turn your hand so that your thumb points forward.

Move your left shoulder back, lift your chin, and arch your back as you slowly lower your arm to your side. Relax.

Do this sequence 3 times with each arm.

the elbow hinge

To get a sense of the muscles of the upper arm in action, locate the elbow hinge.

Sit upright, legs wide apart. Place your right hand, palm up, on your right knee.

Place your left index finger lightly across the inner surface of your right elbow, your thumb on the pointed elbow bone.

Slowly lift your right hand, bending your elbow only slightly. Feel a strong wirelike tendon rising against your index finger, and the pointed elbow bone moving against your thumb.

Resisting the tendency to raise your right shoulder, straighten your right arm by pressing upward at the inner surface of the elbow—as if pushing against that tendon. Feel the muscles in the inner surface of your upper arm tightening.

The tightening of these muscles is your clue that you are activating your elbow joint correctly.

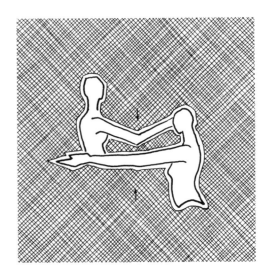

the elbows

The muscles at the inner surfaces of your upper arms are usually idle. Complete articulation of the elbow joint will bring these muscles into play, improving their tone and shape.

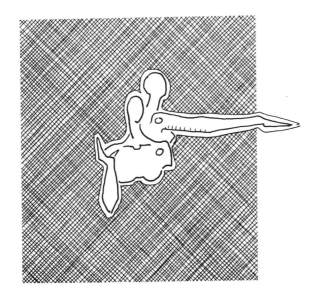

straightening forward

Sit upright, legs wide apart. Place your right thumb against your right shoulder.

Raise your right elbow forward to just below shoulder level. With palm down, and keeping your upper arm and right shoulder still, slowly straighten your arm. Turn your palm up.

Keeping your upper arm still, press downward with your shoulder as you press upward at the inner surface of your elbow.

Feel a strong pull in the inner surface of your upper arm.

Do this 3 times with each arm.

24

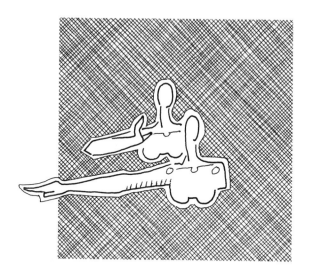

straightening sideways

Sit as before. Place your right thumb against your right shoulder. Raise your elbow to the side, stopping slightly below shoulder level. Keeping your shoulder low, with your palm down and your upper arm still, slowly straighten your arm and press firmly at the elbow. Feel a strong pull in the inner surface of your upper arm.

Do this 3 times with each arm.

straightening backward

Stand upright. Place the back of your right wrist on your right hip, thumb pointing back, elbow akimbo. Keeping your shoulder low, slowly straighten your arm as you move it behind your back. Press firmly at the elbow. Feel a strong pull in the inner surface and along the back of your upper arm.

Do this 3 times with each arm.

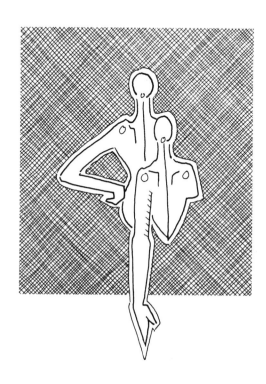

the wrists

Circulation is often poor in the hands. Wrist Articulations will release tension, improve circulation, and make your gestures fluid and graceful.

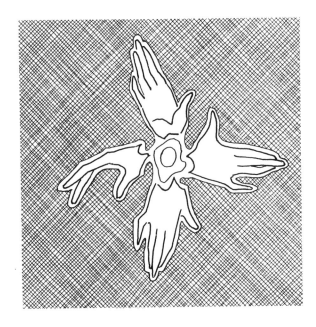

rotating

Sit upright, feet slightly apart. Move your right hand, palm forward, a few inches in front of your chest. Keep your elbow near your side. Relax your wrist and drop your hand as though it were hanging from a thread. Keep your arm as still as possible.
Slowly roll your hand clockwise around the wrist. Pause at the first sign of resistance, relax, then continue to rotate your hand in the largest possible circumference. Relax. Now rotate counterclockwise.

Do this 3 times in each direction, with each hand.

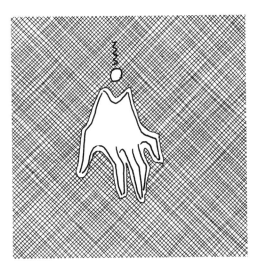

shaking

Sit as before. Brace both elbows against your sides. Drop your wrists limply. Shake your hands gently up and down, then side to side, all for a slow count of 10.
Move your elbows away from your sides; relax your shoulders. Shake your hands more vigorously for a slow count of 10. Raise your arms above your head and hold for a slow count of 10. The tingling sensation in your fingers and palms is due to increased circulation.

Do this sequence once.

the fingers

Finger joints are often the site of the first arthritic changes. The following Articulations will alleviate or prevent stiffness.

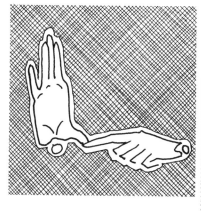

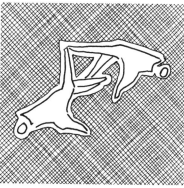

finger pressing

Sit as before. Move your right hand with palm toward you a few inches in front of your chest. Curl your fingers, one at a time, then press them firmly into the fleshy cushions at the top of your palm. Hold for a slow count of 3. Straighten and stretch your fingers. Relax.

Do this 3 times with each hand.

thumb pressing

Sit as before. With palm facing you and fingers straight, move your thumb across your palm. Press your thumb firmly against the base of your little finger. Hold for a slow count of 3.

Do this 3 times with each hand.

thumb stretching

Sit upright, feet slightly apart. Move your right hand, palm forward, in front of your chest. Place your left index finger on the tip of your right thumb. Relax both hands in position. With 6 slow to-and-fro movements, coax your thumb down toward your wrist. Relax.

Do this 3 times with each hand.

finger stretching

Sit as before. Move your right hand, palm down, in front of your chest, your right elbow slightly to the side. Raise your right index finger slightly and put your left index finger against its tip. Relax both hands in position. With 6 slow to-and-fro movements coax your right finger up and away from the palm. Relax. Stretch each finger in the same manner.

Do this 3 times with each hand.

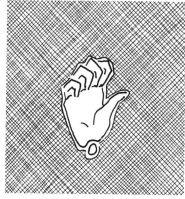

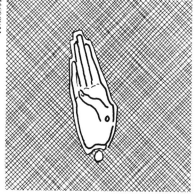

spine and shoulder girdle

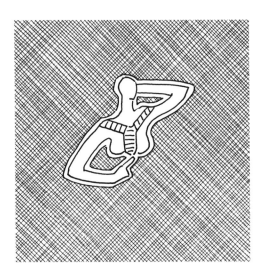

spine and diaphragm

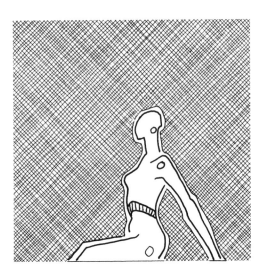

Your spine and your shoulder girdle interact. Sit upright. Place your right index finger at the base of your breastbone and the fingers of your left hand across the back of your neck. Slump by lowering your breastbone. Feel the position of your neck changing. Lift upward with the back of your neck. Feel your breastbone rising. Lift and lower until you are familiar with these interactions.

Chronic tension in the area of your diaphragm—a dome-shaped muscle partition that divides your chest from your abdominal area—deprives the spine of mobility and the body of an adequate oxygen supply. "Holding your stomach in" contributes to the worst kind of body tension. When we breathe, our diaphragm acts as a bellows; when we are tense and our diaphragm is rigid, breathing is shallow and often irregular. The following Articulations will help to relax the diaphragm area and the spine. Don't be reluctant to relax your abdominal wall. The Posture Toning movements in Part 2 will strengthen the muscles that keep your abdominal wall firm and flat.

the diaphragm

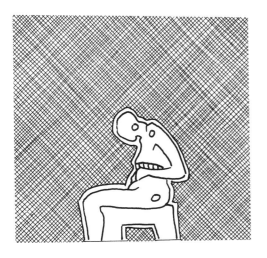

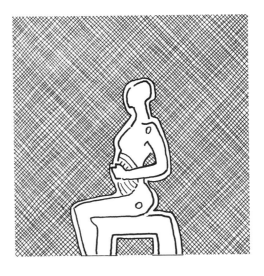

relaxing

Place both hands high on your abdomen and slump. Lower your head. Do not allow your chest to lift as you slowly and deeply inhale and exhale. Feel your abdomen expanding as you inhale and deflating as you exhale.

Do this 3 times.

expanding

Sit upright, hands high on your abdomen. Move your elbows to the sides, then press them back firmly as you arch your back. Inhale and exhale deeply. Feel your abdomen expanding as you inhale and deflating as you exhale. Resume your starting position.

Do this 3 times.

the spine

The spine, because of its limited mobility, is particularly prone to tension. Move very slowly and with great care during spine Articulations, and remain relaxed.

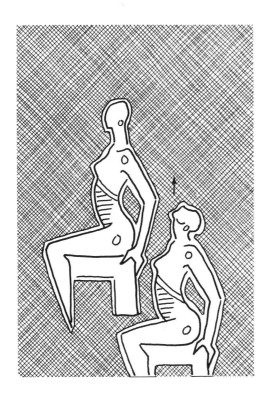

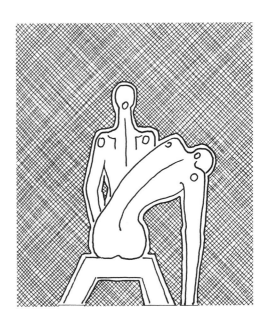

arching

Sit slightly forward in your chair, feet apart, hands holding the chair near your hips. Lift your rib cage and gently let your spine arch, without straining. Lift your chin and move your shoulders back to increase the arching. Relax and resume your starting position.

Do this 3 times.

curving sideways

Sit upright, legs wide apart, arms relaxed at your sides. Place your left hand on your right knee, fingers pointing forward. Lift your left shoulder and straighten your left arm. Bend slowly sideways to the right as if you were reaching for something on the floor, but only as far as comfort will allow. Move slowly upward to center. Relax.

Do this 3 times on each side.

arching in rotation

Sit upright and slightly forward in your chair, legs wide apart. Move your right hand, palm out, and place it against your left hip. Put your left hand on your right shoulder.

Remain in this rotated position. Move your right hand forward and cup it under your left elbow.

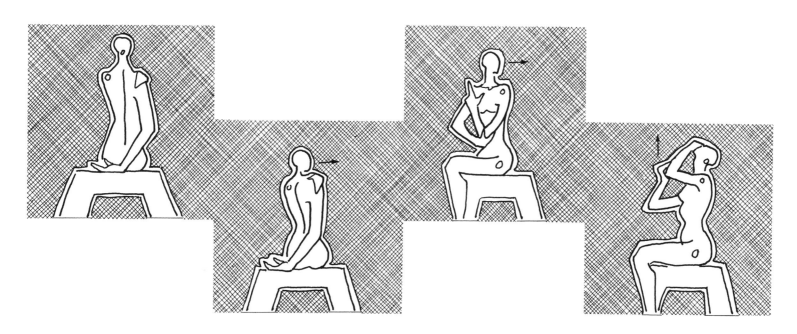

Turn your head and look over your right shoulder, as you turn your shoulders as far to the right as comfort will allow.

Raise your rib cage, then slowly raise both arms to above shoulder level. Roll your head back as you arch your back. Resume starting position. Feel a release of tension along your back.

Do this sequence 3 times on each side.

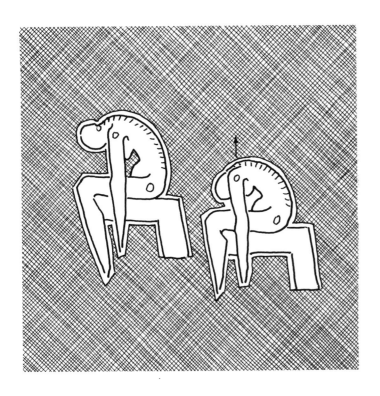

curving forward

Sit upright, feet slightly apart, arms relaxed at your sides. Lower your head and shoulders. Lift your chin slightly. <u>Slowly and carefully</u> bend forward and down, curving your spine. Lower your chin toward your chest and lift your shoulders. <u>Feel your spine stretching.</u> Lower your shoulders and sit upright.

Do this 3 times.

the hip joints

Your hip joints rotate freely. The ball-shaped head of the thighbone fits into a cup-shaped cavity in the hipbone. This cavity is lined with a membrane that secretes a lubricating substance, which allows virtually frictionless articulation.

forward lift

With the back of a chair at your left, stand upright, feet apart and slightly turned out. Place your left hand on the back of the chair. Slowly lift—<u>do not kick</u>—your right knee toward your chest, allowing your left knee to bend. Bend down slightly toward your right knee. Lower your right leg; stand straight.

Do this 4 times on each side.

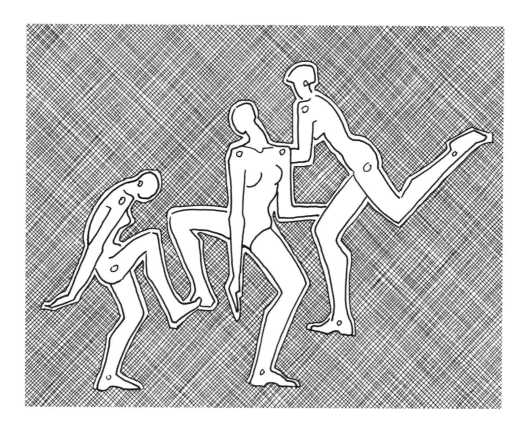

side lift

Stand with feet slightly apart and well turned out. Place your left hand on the back of your chair. With your right arm straight down in front of your body, slowly lift your right knee to the side, aiming it behind your shoulder, allowing your left knee to bend. Lower your right leg; stand straight.

Do this 4 times on each side.

back lift

Stand with feet slightly turned out. Face your chair and place both hands on its back. Lean slightly forward. Bend your left knee and move it directly back and up from the hip joint as far as comfort allows, keeping your foot relaxed and allowing your right knee to bend. Lower your left leg; straighten both legs. Feel the easy, rolling motions of the hip joint.

Do this 4 times on each side.

the knees

Your knees are shock absorbers. Because they are seldom fully articulated, they tend to be tense and are prone to localized fat deposits. The shape of your inner thighs is improved by the thorough Articulation of your knee joints.

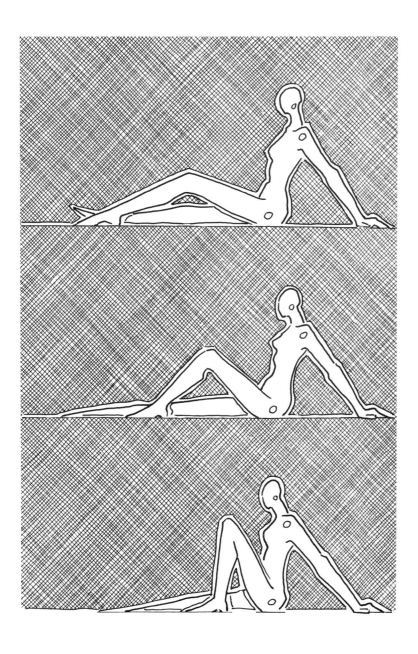

slight bending

Sit on the floor, legs straight and slightly separated. Place your hands at a comfortable distance behind your back. Do not let your knees turn out. Bend your left knee and place your foot flat on the floor, aligning the toes with your right ankle. Keep your foot flat; don't let the toes curl up. Lift your rib cage by arching your back and slowly move it forward. Relax.

Do this 3 times with each leg.

increased bending

Sit as before. Bend your left knee and place your foot flat on the floor, aligning the arch with your right knee. Lift your rib cage by arching your back and slowly move it forward. Relax.

Do this 3 times with each leg.

maximal bending

Sit as before. Bend your left knee and place your foot flat on the floor, as close to the buttock as possible. Lift your rib cage by arching your back and slowly move it forward. Relax.

Do this 3 times with each leg.

the ankles

Ankle joints are often stiff and tense, although you may not realize it. Tension in these joints inhibits movement of the calf muscles and reduces circulation. Furthermore, this area has great potential for stimulating circulation throughout your body, for in each calf muscle is a special vein, like a small pumping mechanism. As the calf muscle contracts in response to ankle movement, this "pump" squeezes blood through the veins toward the heart. As the calf muscle relaxes, the veins open to receive more blood.

If your feet are not in good condition, repeat the following Articulations later in the day, preferably at bedtime. This will relax not only your feet but your entire body as well.

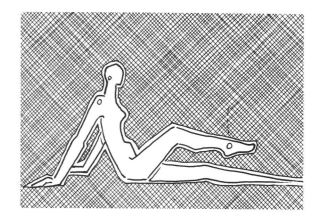

shaking

Sit on the floor with legs straight. Place your hands at a comfortable distance behind your back. Lift your right leg and let your foot dangle, as if it were hanging by a thread. Shake your foot gently for a slow count of 10.

Do this once with each ankle.

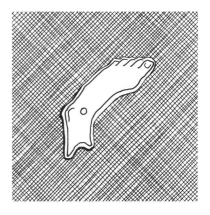

turning in

Sit as before. Place your legs about 12 inches apart. Without allowing your legs to move, turn your ankles slowly inward as far as possible. Hold to the count of 3, then move your ankles back to starting position.

Do this 6 times.

flexing

Sit on the floor, legs straight and slightly separated. Place your hands at a comfortable distance behind your back. Do not allow your knees to turn out. Relax your ankles; then slowly slide your heels forward until your feet are at right angles to your legs. Do not force. Relax and return to your starting position.

Do this 4 times.

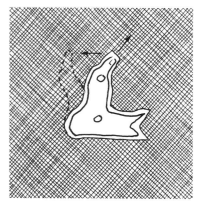

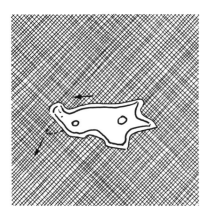

arching

Sit as before. Plan to keep your toes relaxed. Moving from the ankles, slowly slide your heels back toward the calves, then reach toward the floor with your toes. Relax. Return to your starting position.

Do this 4 times.

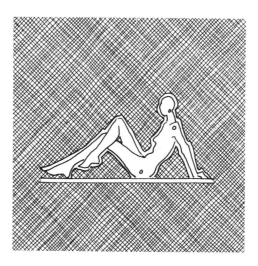

rotating

Sit as before. Bend both knees and cross your right leg over your left leg, letting your right foot dangle. Slowly rotate your right foot in as complete a circle as possible, first clockwise, then counterclockwise.

Do this 3 times with each foot.

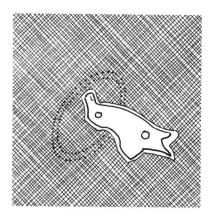

the toes

Toe Articulations activate the muscles of your lower legs. The tendons of your small toes unite in a large tendon at your instep, near your outer anklebone; this in turn connects with a muscle you can feel along the outer side of your shinbone when you flex your toes.

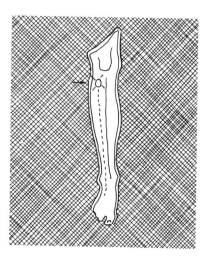 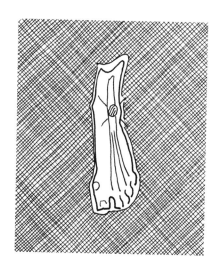

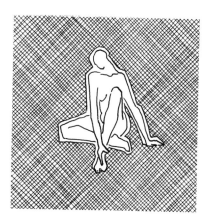

Sit on the floor, with your right leg tucked under your left thigh. Bend your left knee and place your foot flat on the floor. Rest your right index finger lightly on the area marked "X" in the illustration. Keeping the ball of your left foot on the floor, slowly and firmly press your toes upward. Feel the wirelike tendon rising toward your finger. Relax. Repeat with your right foot.

To avoid cramps, move slowly and gently during all Toe Articulations, and make sure to relax completely after each effort.

Discomfort in tense, neglected toes will reflect in your face and affect your health and disposition. Toe Articulations will help to release tensions and lend spring to your step.

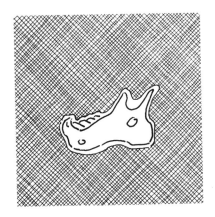

flexing

Sit on the floor, legs straight in front, and place your hands at a comfortable distance behind your back. Bend your knees and put your feet flat on the floor.

Slowly press your toes upward; try to include your little toes in the effort. Hold to a slow count of 3. Relax. If some toes fail to respond, use your finger to coax them upward until they can move without your aid.

Do this 6 times.

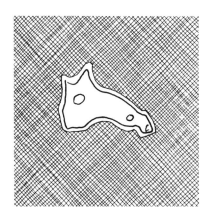

curling

Sit as before. Keeping your heels on the floor, lift your feet at least 1 inch off the floor. Slowly curl your toes under as far as possible. Hold for a slow count of 3, then lower your curled toes to the floor. Relax.

Do this 6 times.

grasping

Sit upright on the floor, right leg tucked under your left thigh. Bend your left knee and place your left foot flat on the floor. Slide a pen or pencil under all five toes. Curl your toes around it and grasp firmly. Hold for a slow count of 5. Relax.

Do this 3 times with each foot.

big toe lifts

This is the toe that gives you push-off power in walking.

Sit as before. Place your fingers lightly on the four small toes of your left foot to keep them from rising. Gently and without forcing, attempt to lift and lower only the big toe. Relax after each attempt.

Do this 6 times with each foot.

When you have succeeded in lifting the big toe without holding the others down, ...

Do this 6 times with each foot.

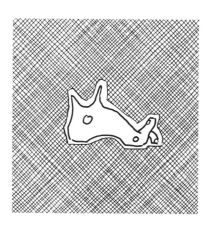

small toe lifts

Sit as before. Place your left index finger on the big toe of your right foot. Do not allow this toe to lift. With the ball of your foot on the floor, lift only the small toes. Hold for a count of 3. Relax.

Do this 6 times with each foot.

When you have succeeded in lifting the small toes without holding the big toe, ...

Do this 6 times with each foot.

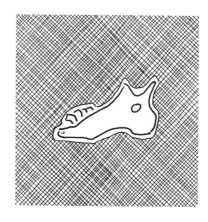

tension brakes

The new freedom and relaxation you derive from practicing Articulations will not remain with you for long unless you carry what you have learned into your work and play. The less you move, the greater your potential for tension and nerve fatigue. Nerve cells tire not only from physical and mental work, but also from monotony of movement—from lack of stimulation. A variety of movement calls different muscle groups into play, which refreshes your nervous system.

Make it a habit, while shopping or on your way to work, to walk in your normal fashion for 20 steps, then alternate between 20 somewhat longer steps, 20 shorter steps, and 20 normal steps. After changing the length of your steps for a while, change your speed every 20 steps.

To counteract the ill effects of the sedentary existence so many of us lead, and to put a brake on tensions that are bound to accumulate in the course of a day, keep your body active in small and unobtrusive ways. Above all, don't shrug off the subtle warning signals that precede tension.

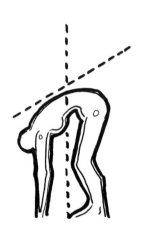

Are you aware of yourself at this moment? Are your hands and shoulders relaxed as you hold this book? Are your jaws tensed, and are you frowning in concentration? Tensions like these set up a chain reaction that affects your facial muscles. Aren't we all familiar with the strained, anxious expressions of tense people?

To counteract tensions, try these simple innovations. Don't grip a telephone receiver; keep your hand relaxed. If you are right-handed, use your left hand more often. As you work at a desk, table, or sewing machine, try to keep your feet and ankles moving. Periodically curl your toes under and relax them again; you can do this even with shoes on. Shift your position in your chair, and from time to time move your chair closer to your work surface, then farther away.

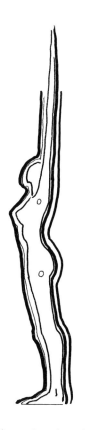

Arch your back frequently. Always turn your head a little farther than needed. Lengthen the back of your neck often and adjust your shoulders, keeping them low and relaxed.

If you work at an ironing board or counter, take time out to rotate your shoulders and to bend your knees several times.

When you comb or brush your hair, remember to activate the weak muscles in the inner surface of your upper arm. Place small articles of clothing on a high shelf, so that you will have to stretch in order to reach them.

Whenever you have a moment of privacy, open your mouth wide and pretend that you are yawning. Lift and lower your eyebrows firmly and make an effort to relax the muscles in your forehead.

Inhale and exhale deeply from time to time.
And smile! Nothing so refreshes and tones the facial muscles as a friendly grin.

Use your imagination. Invent new ways of doing familiar things and you'll soon feel more relaxed and alert.

Posture

posture and gravity

Posture is your dynamic signature. It is what allows others to recognize you in a crowd or at a distance, although they may see no more of you than the silhouette of your receding back. However you project yourself—as a person of significance or as one lacking in self-assurance—your posture is a clue to your personality and a vital part of the image you present to the world.

The first steps in infancy—though celebrated as a great triumph—commit you to the lifelong effort of keeping your body upright and balanced against the constant earthward force of gravity, a force that determines your needs as a structural entity for stability, mobility, power, and control. Even as you stand, apparently at ease, your body is never entirely still. Your balance as a vertical, multijointed, and flexible structure, poised on a base of support that is relatively small in relation to its height, is a product of reflexes—a series of continuous minute adjustments to the pull of gravity. And while you may be unconscious of this in yourself, you can see it clearly in the constant swaying of a public speaker.

To appreciate how your body relates to gravity's pull, think of it as a segmented column.

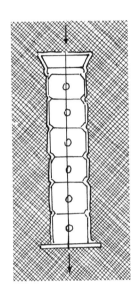

A mark in the center of each segment indicates its center of weight, or center of gravity.

A vertical line passing through these marks is the line of gravity.

Though this line is invisible, it represents a very real force: the power and direction of gravitational pull.

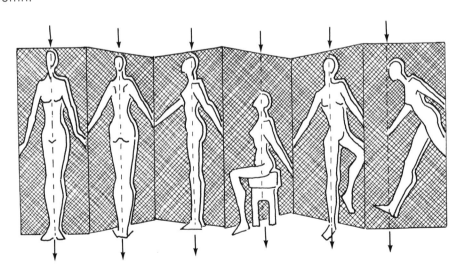

The line of gravity passes through the body, to its base of support.

Usually you are not aware of the downward pull of gravity, but you feel its effect when you are tired and become unpleasantly conscious of your body's weight. Whether you experience your body as a burden or as an instrument of buoyancy depends upon the quality of your posture.

Three factors apply when you evaluate your posture: how it looks, how it feels, and how much energy it demands. Poor posture, by freely yielding to gravity, appears to demand the least energy, but you pay a price in looks and, in the long run, in health and feeling. Certain postures that at first glance look impressive, are actually forced and rigid, and their cost in energy is enormous.

The militaristic formula for posture (Shoulders back! Chest out! Stomach in!) is frankly outdated. Good posture consists of a happy compromise—it enhances appearance and promotes a feeling of well-being without undue expenditure of energy.

Poor posture damages you physically and psychologically. Misalignment—which causes uneven pressure on ligaments and abnormal friction in joints—is a major cause of back pain and of tensions that sap your energy. Poor circulation and inadequate oxygen intake—caused by rounded shoulders and a depressed chest—lower your vitality. And because your sense of well-being is so closely linked to your vitality level, poor posture invites depression and delivers you into a limbo of chronic aches and pains that guarantee premature aging.

Fortunately, posture can be improved in simple, basic ways. The shape and performance of your body depend almost entirely on its interior frame—your skeletal structure—and the most lasting physical improvements are based on its correct alignment.

Your body is well-aligned, or well-centered, when the center of gravity of each body segment is poised directly above the center of gravity of the segment beneath, and when the line of gravity falls within the area of the base of its support.

Your body is misaligned when any segment deviates from the line of gravity. Although poor postures occur in many variations, any misalignment is always balanced by an equal misalignment in the opposite direction. For every zig there is a zag.

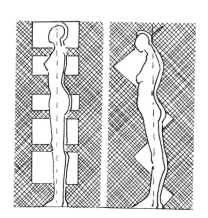

Correct alignment will stabilize your body and minimize the wearing effects of gravity's pull. That is why trying to improve your posture without first correcting alignment is like recovering a chair without first repairing its broken springs. No amount of surface adjustment will make it support you in comfort or improve its shape. Good shapes are built from inside out.

By following the techniques outlined in this program, you can develop an attractive, efficient posture, regardless of your physique, age, heredity, or habits.

The rewards will astonish you. A well-aligned body often increases up to two inches in height, and enjoys better circulation and a greater capacity for oxygen intake. The sum of these benefits is a marked improvement in health and appearance, and an exhilarating gain in vitality.

Posture training is not limited to alignment and to the strengthening of support muscles. It includes memorizing the varied sensations that accompany postural adjustments.

You may not have thought of physical training in terms of memorizing sensations, but that is exactly how athletes perfect their skills. Good posture, which is also an acquired skill, requires the same attention to small and delicate adjustments.

Visualize with what precision a golfer patiently adjusts and readjusts the position of his feet. Or the hair-trigger alertness with which a tennis player crouches to estimate the direction and force of a moving ball. It is a highly developed kinesthetic sense that will make you a champion, whether you are a golfer or a tennis star, or whether you simply stand and move like one.

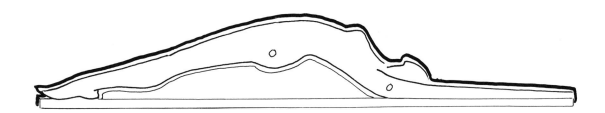

Alignments

This portion of your posture training is devoted to Alignments, the structural adjustments that produce good posture, and to body awareness, the sensitivity to sensory information by which you determine how your body is and should be aligned.

Although Alignments are practiced in segments, every part of your body is related to every other, and each partial adjustment will contribute to your total alignment.

Practice in front of a full-length mirror, wearing little clothing. Relax, and concentrate on your sensations. Control the degree of your efforts. Alignments require very small adjustments—measuring no more than inches, and at times only fractions of inches.

Alignments are practiced in the following order:

1) The Soles and Ankles
2) The Knees
3) The Pelvis
4) The Spine
5) The Shoulders
6) The Neck and Head

program

"Once each" may mean once each, or once on each side, or once in each direction, whichever applies.

1) Practice for 2 days:

All Articulations, once each.

All Alignments, all repeats.

2) Practice for 2 days:

All Articulations, once each.

All Alignments, once each.

If poor posture is your main problem, continue to practice Alignments for several additional days.

the soles and ankles

Well-aligned feet and ankles are fundamental to good body architecture. Correct alignment of your ankles depends upon the correct distribution of weight on the soles of your feet.

o To counteract the pull of gravity, carry your weight mainly on the balls of your feet, letting your heels serve their function as shock absorbers.

o Bearing down on your heels will prevent your spine from straightening completely.

Stand upright, facing your mirror, arms relaxed, feet slightly apart and slightly turned out. Concentrate on the distribution of your weight along the length of your soles; on the distribution of your weight across the width of your soles; and on the positioning of your ankles.

a) Do you habitually carry your weight on your heels?

b) Do you carry your weight well forward on the balls of your feet?

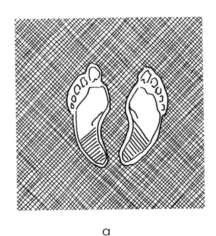

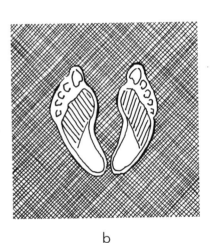

a b

TO DISTRIBUTE YOUR WEIGHT CORRECTLY ALONG THE LENGTH OF YOUR SOLES, stand as above.

a) Without allowing your heels to lift, or your spine to move in the slightest degree, slowly shift your weight forward until it rests mainly on the balls of your feet. Hold this position for a slow count of 5.
Feel the muscles along the backs of your legs tightening.

b) Without allowing your toes to lift, or your spine to move in the slightest degree, slowly shift your weight back along your soles until it rests mainly on your heels.
Feel the muscles of your upper back, and those above your knees and along the front of your thighs, slackening.

c) Slowly shift your weight forward again until it rests on the balls of your feet.

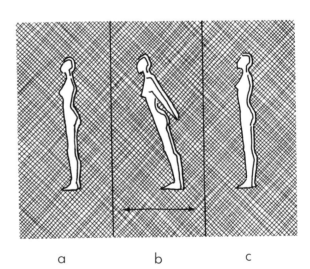

a b c

Do this sequence 6 times.

48

Correct distribution of your weight across the width of your soles will stabilize your ankles, make you sure-footed, and encourage an even distribution of effort in the muscles of your feet, ankles, and legs.

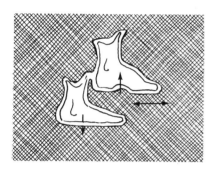

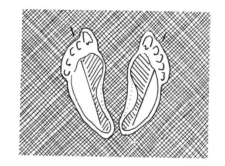

a

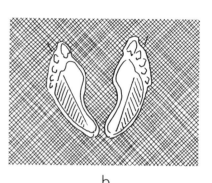

b

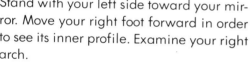

Stand with your left side toward your mirror. Move your right foot forward in order to see its inner profile. Examine your right arch.

Is your arch clearly defined?

Does it appear flattened?

Is your inner anklebone close to the floor?

Face your mirror, arms relaxed, feet slightly apart and parallel.
Visualize the surface of your soles.

a) Do you place more weight on their inner half?

b) Do you place more weight on their outer half?

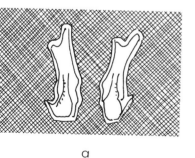

a

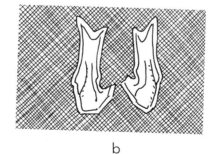

b

Do this sequence 6 times.

TO DISTRIBUTE YOUR WEIGHT ACROSS THE WIDTH OF YOUR SOLES CORRECTLY, IN ORDER TO ALIGN YOUR ANKLES, stand as above. Plan to keep your knees perfectly straight.

a) Roll your ankles inward. Stop.

b) Roll your ankles out until your weight rests on the outer rims of your soles. Stop. Slowly distribute your weight evenly across the width of your soles.
Feel your ankles aligning, and your arches lifting slightly, as you shift your weight forward to the balls of your feet.

49

the knees

Correct alignment of your knees will help to align your pelvis and improve the shape of your legs. Knees require alignment from two aspects: from in <u>front</u> and in <u>profile</u>.

Stand with your right side toward your mirror, arms relaxed, heels together, feet slightly turned out. Examine your legs.

a) Are your knees hyperextended?

b) Do they jut forward, making your kneecaps appear prominent and angular?

c) Do your knees conform to the line of gravity?

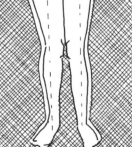

Misalignment of the knees often makes it appear that the shape of the legs is faulty. In most cases, the correct alignment of the knees will help to straighten the legs.

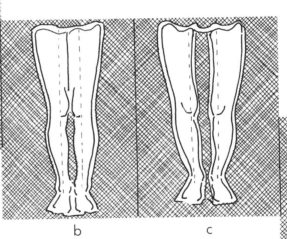

Stand facing your mirror, arms relaxed, heels together, feet slightly turned out.

a) Visualize the line of gravity along the front of your legs.

b) Are your kneecaps centered on this line, or do they turn inward?

c) Do your legs appear to be bowed?

d) Do your feet extend sideways, beyond your knees?

TO ALIGN YOUR KNEES CORRECTLY IN PROFILE, stand as above.

a) With your weight on the balls of your feet, and without lifting your heels, bend and separate your knees slightly. Keep your torso upright.

b) Allowing your spine to curve, tilt your pelvis under and forward.

c) Pressing firmly forward at the insteps, slowly straighten your legs until they conform to the line of gravity.

If your knees are hyperextended, avoid any pressure whatsoever at the back of your knees as you straighten your legs. Should you find that your kneecaps still appear unduly prominent, press very firmly backward at the back of your knees as you straighten your legs.

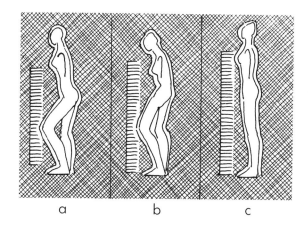

a   b   c

Do this sequence 6 times, according to your needs.

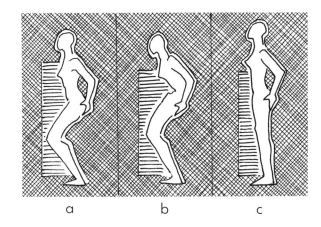

a   b   c

Do this sequence 8 times, resting after each effort.

TO ALIGN YOUR KNEES CORRECTLY FROM IN FRONT, YOU MUST WORK FROM THE HIP JOINTS. Stand as above. Plan to keep your weight on the balls of your feet, without allowing your heels to lift.

a) Keeping your torso upright, bend and separate your knees slightly.

b) Place your hands on the sides of your buttocks. Allow your spine to curve as you tilt your pelvis under and forward.

c) Turn your thighs out as far as possible as you straighten your legs. Feel your buttocks and thigh muscles tightening, and your knees aligning.

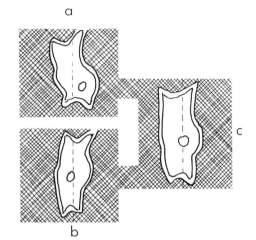

the pelvis

The shape of your body is tremendously influenced by the position of your pelvis. When your pelvis is aligned correctly, your abdominal muscles perform like a firm natural girdle.

TO ALIGN YOUR PELVIS CORRECTLY, stand as above. Without tensing your shoulders, lengthen the back of your neck. Raise your rib cage slightly. Plan to keep your legs perfectly straight and still.

Stand facing your mirror, feet slightly apart and slightly turned out. Raise your rib cage and, without lowering your chin, place your hands lightly on top of your head. Examine the position of your pelvis.

a) Is it tilted back too far?

b) Do you stand hipshot, with your pelvis slanting forward?

c) Is your pelvis centered on the line of gravity?

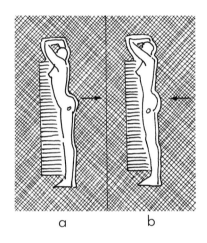

a) Slowly tilt your pelvis back as far as possible, without straining.

b) Raising your rib cage, tilt your pelvis under and forward until it is centered on the line of gravity. Hold this position for a slow count of 3. Relax. Feel a strong contraction in your buttocks and thigh muscles and a firm flattening of your abdominal wall.

Do this sequence 6 times.

the spine

Your spine is a segmented, flexible column, not unlike a series of beads strung on an elastic band. To prevent your spine from overreacting during alignment, move slowly and carefully.

Stand with your side toward the mirror, arms relaxed, heels together, feet slightly turned out. Examine your spine.

a) Is your back rounded?

b) Does your lower back show a pronounced arch?

c) Does your spine conform to the line of gravity?

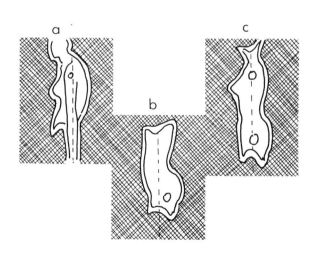

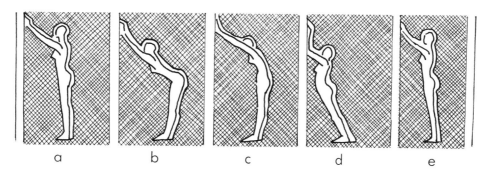

a b c d e

TO ALIGN YOUR SPINE CORRECTLY, stand facing a wall, heels together, feet slightly turned out. Lift your arms above your head and place your hands on the wall, a shoulders' width apart.

a) Step back two short paces.

b) Relax your shoulders and arch your back as you move your hips back as far as possible.

c) Raise your shoulders and allow your spine to curve as you tilt your pelvis under and forward. Feel the increased length of your spine.

d) Relax and lower your shoulders. Straighten your back and, bending your elbow, slowly move your abdomen toward the wall until your spine is fully arched.

e) As you resume an upright position, lengthen your spine and conform to the line of gravity by aligning the back of your head with your shoulder blades, hips, calves, and heels.

Do this sequence 4 times.

the shoulders

Instead of consciously "carrying" your shoulders, keep them low and relaxed. Correct alignment of your shoulders—which depends mainly on the correct alignment of your spine—will allow your neck to rise gracefully and free from tensions.

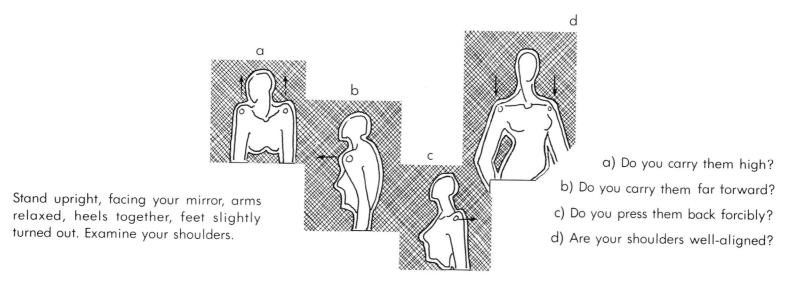

Stand upright, facing your mirror, arms relaxed, heels together, feet slightly turned out. Examine your shoulders.

a) Do you carry them high?

b) Do you carry them far torward?

c) Do you press them back forcibly?

d) Are your shoulders well-aligned?

53

TO ALIGN YOUR SHOULDERS CORRECTLY, stand as above and <u>concentrate on the weight of your arms.</u>

a) Without allowing your spine to curve, slowly raise your shoulders as high as possible.

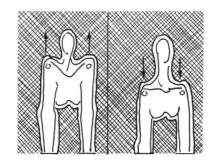

b) Without allowing your shoulders to move back in the slightest degree, slowly lower your shoulders and, pressing firmly downward with your hands, lengthen the back of your neck.

Do this sequence 6 times.

the neck and head

The positioning of your neck—which determines the alignment of your head—greatly influences your posture, your looks, and your sense of well-being. Misalignment of your neck increases the gravity pull on your head, making it feel heavy. A firm chin line and smooth neck depend upon the correct alignment of your head.

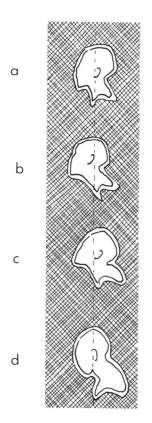

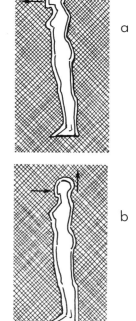

Stand upright, facing your mirror, arms relaxed, heels together, feet slightly turned out. Examine the position of your neck and head.

a) Is your head well-aligned?

b) Do you carry your head too far forward?

c) Do you habitually lift your chin?

d) Do you habitually lower your chin?

TO ALIGN YOUR NECK AND HEAD CORRECTLY, stand as above.

a) Keeping your body still, and resisting the impulse to move your shoulders forward, slowly move your chin forward as far as possible. <u>Feel your neck lengthening along a horizontal plane.</u>

b) Slowly, and without pressing, move your head upward from the atlas as you slide your chin back until your neck is fully extended. Relax.

Do this sequence 6 times.

Posture Toning

This portion of your program is designed primarily to strengthen the muscles that make sustained good alignment possible. And since your muscles operate in sets of relationships, the movements in this section will also help to shape your body.

During this part of your training, concentrate on perceiving the subtlest sensations, move slowly and deliberately, and use only as much energy as each movement requires. What counts in this training is not the force but the precision with which you work. If at first you feel strain or fatigue in your legs, stop and shake them vigorously before proceeding.

program

"Once each" may mean once each, or once on each side, or once in each direction, whichever applies.

1)   Practice for 2 days:

All Articulations, once each.

Posture Toning 1 to 6, all repeats.

2)   Practice for 2 days:

All Articulations, once each.

Posture Toning 1 to 6, once each.

Posture Toning 7 to 9, all repeats.

3)   Practice for 2 days:

All Articulations, once each.

Posture Toning 1 to 9, once each.

Memorize Posture Toning 7, 8 and 9.

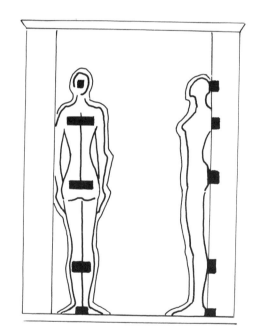

To begin the movements in Posture Toning, stand upright with your back against a flush surface, either a flush door or a wall. A protruding baseboard should not present a problem. Make a 5-point contact with this surface at 1) your heels, 2) your calves, 3) your buttocks, 4) your shoulder blades, and 5) the back of your head.

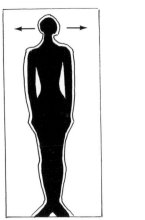

1

Stand in 5-point contact, arms relaxed, heels together, feet slightly turned out. Keeping your head in contact with the wall, and without straining, slowly turn your head as far as possible toward the right, then toward the left. Relax. Resume your starting position.

Do this 4 times.

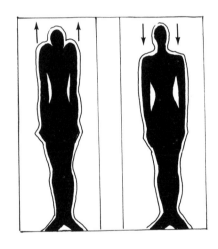

2

Stand as before. Keeping your arms relaxed and your shoulder blades in contact with the wall, slowly raise your shoulders as high as possible. Pressing firmly downward, slowly lower them.

Do this 4 times.

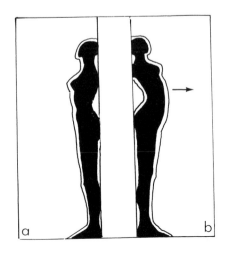

3

a) Stand as before. With your arms straight, place your palms against the wall.

b) With your head and buttocks remaining against the wall, press back with your palms as you arch your back by moving your chest forward, but only as far as comfort will allow. Relax and resume your starting position.

Do this 4 times.

4
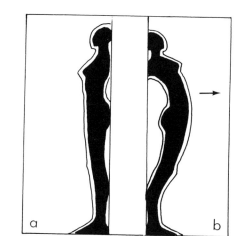

a) Stand as before, keeping your head and calves against the wall.

b) Arch your back by moving both your chest and hips forward as you press firmly back with your palms. Relax. Resume your starting position.

Do this 4 times.

5
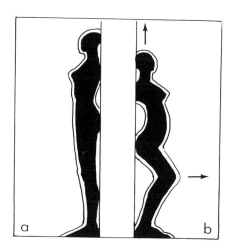

a) Stand as before, arms relaxed along your sides. Plan to keep your weight on the balls of your feet, and do not allow your heels to lift.

b) Keeping your torso upright, bend and separate your knees slightly. Exert a mild pressure toward center at the inner surfaces of your upper thighs as you slowly straighten your legs.
Feel a strong contraction in the muscles of your upper thighs, buttocks, and lower abdomen. As you resume your starting position, try to position your knees on the gravity line.

Do this 4 times.

6

a) Stand as before. Plan to keep your weight on the balls of your feet, and do not allow your heels to lift.

b) Keeping your torso upright, bend and separate your knees slightly more than before.

c) Allow your spine to curve as you slowly tilt your pelvis under and forward. Lower your chin toward your chest.

d) Exert a mild pressure toward center at the inner surfaces of your calves as you slowly straighten your legs.

Feel a strong pull in the muscles of the buttocks, hips, thighs, and lower legs, and a powerful contraction of the abdominal wall. Relax. Resume your starting position and shake your legs thoroughly.

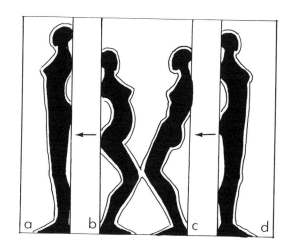

Do this sequence 4 times.

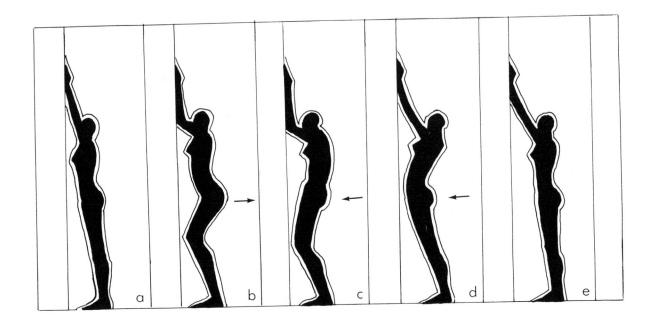

7   Stand facing the wall a foot away, heels together, feet slightly turned out.

a) Raise your arms overhead and place your hands on the wall, shoulders' width apart.

b) Arch your back and, moving your hips well back, bend and separate your knees deeply enough for your elbows to touch the wall.

c) Keeping your ankles steady, allow your spine to curve as you slowly tilt your pelvis under and forward.

d) Keeping your pelvis in the forward position, slowly straighten your legs. Relax. Arching your back, move your abdomen forward toward the wall, but only as far as comfort will allow. Feel a powerful stretch along your legs and through your entire body.

e) Conform to the line of gravity as you resume position a).

Do this sequence once.

Repeat this sequence, once each time, in the following variations:
1)   with feet 8 inches apart and parallel.
2)   with feet 8 inches apart and turned out well.

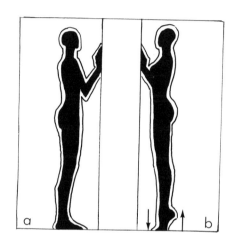

8 a) Stand facing the wall, a foot away, heels together, feet slightly turned out. Plan to keep your knees perfectly straight and your weight on the balls of your feet.

Place your hands on the wall at shoulder level, shoulders' width apart.

b) Tighten your buttock muscles and press firmly downward on your toes as you lift your heels. Heels together, keep your weight mainly on your big toes. Without allowing your spine to arch or your knees to bend, tilt your pelvis gently under and forward, until you feel your abdominal muscles contracting. Feel a powerful contraction in the muscles of your buttocks, thighs, and calves.

Keep your weight well forward on the balls of your feet as you slowly lower your heels to the floor. Relax. Shake your legs thoroughly.

Do this sequence 3 times.

Repeat this sequence, 3 times each, in the following variations:
1) with feet 6 inches apart and parallel.
2) with feet 6 inches apart and slightly turned in.

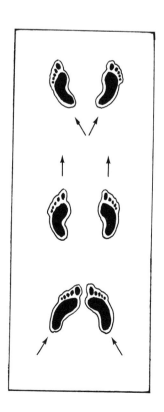

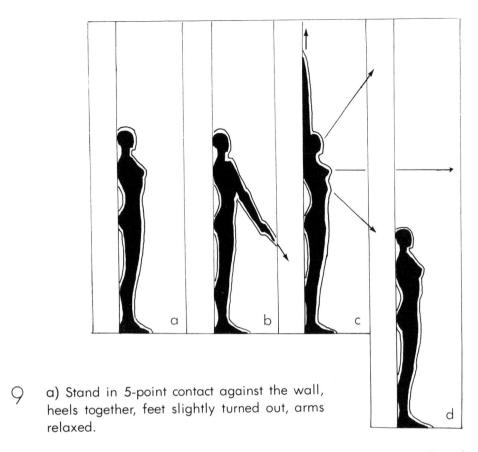

9   a) Stand in 5-point contact against the wall, heels together, feet slightly turned out, arms relaxed.

b) Stiffen your arms. Maintain a steady pressure in your arms and hands as you slowly raise them forward, stopping slightly below shoulder level.

c) Without tensing your shoulders, lift your rib cage and continue to press your arms upward until they are above your head and touching the wall. Relax in position. Inhale and exhale deeply.
Without forcing, move your hands upward along the wall until your body is stretched to full capacity. Concentrate on your increased length and retain it as you stiffen your arms, then move them away from the wall.

d) With the same steady pressure as before, slowly lower your arms, thumbs up, to shoulder level. Stop. Lower your shoulders and gradually, with continued pressure, lower your arms to your sides. Relax completely. Shake your legs.

Do this sequence once.

Repeat once each in the following variations:
1)   with feet 6 inches apart and parallel.
2)   with feet 6 inches apart and slightly turned in.

about your back

Although your posture training has strengthened your back muscles, strength in itself is no guarantee against back pain and related problems. To prevent back problems you must learn to protect your back.

<u>Begin by attending to your feet.</u> Even the smallest callus or corn, by making you shift your weight away from local pain, can ruin your alignment. Discard ill-fitting shoes, no matter how pretty or expensive. A recent generation of women grew up believing that tiny feet were beautiful and all but crippled themselves; even though we no longer believe such nonsense, we are rarely careful enough about choosing the correct last and shoe size. Feet continue to grow, so have them measured each time you buy shoes, and make sure that your stockings don't bind your toes.

If you have painful corns or calluses or pronounced bunions, by all means seek professional help. If you have only a hint of a bunion, practice toe-pulling and articulate your big toes with special care. Move your big toes, not from the tip end, but from the joint, where the metatarsal and toe bones meet.

Slowly and gently pull your big toes, one at a time, at least 10 times before going to bed, and rotate them a little before releasing the pull.

To protect your back, pay attention to how you move. There are right and wrong ways to sit, move, lift, bend, and stretch. You may recall our mentioning, on page 5, how frequently people try to touch their toes by bending, not from the hip joints, which would make it easier for them, but from the small of the back, which makes the movement more difficult and may be harmful.

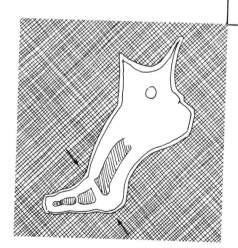

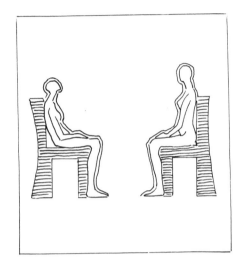

Whenever you have a choice, head for a straight-backed chair. Sitting correctly will protect the delicate area around the base of your spine from undue strain.

Keep your back straight and bend your knees when you pick something up from the floor.

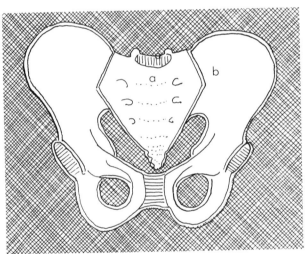

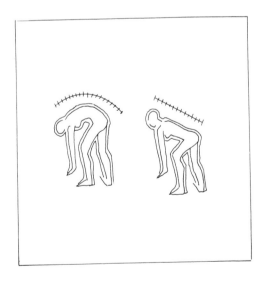

The sacrum, a triangular, bony plate, is wedged between your hipbones at the lower back. Your spine rises from an indentation in its upper part (a), not unlike a candle in a candlestick. This is the place to watch out for when you move; most problems start here, although you may feel pain in the areas indicated (b).

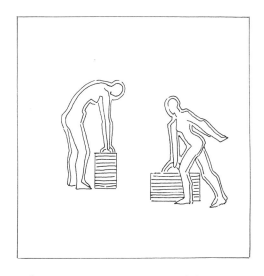

When you lift a heavy suitcase, stand at its side and close to its center. Place your feet about 10 inches apart, then step forward with the foot farther away from the suitcase. Bend both knees slightly and, with your back straight, reach for its handle with a perfectly straight arm. Protect your back by using the power in your legs as you straighten up and lift it.

When you move a piece of furniture, always place your hands at the center of its height and stand at a distance from it with both arms at full length. Place one foot behind the other and brace your whole weight against the object, using your weight and the power in your legs to move it. When you take something off a high shelf, stand at some distance from the shelf and place one foot behind the other for good balance.

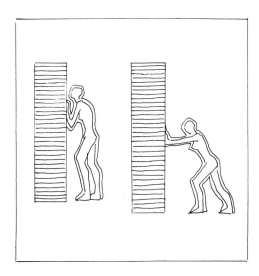

Above all, apply the principles of good alignment throughout the day. No one will notice a slight tensing of your buttocks, so practice aligning your knees and pelvis as you stand at a counter or wait for a bus. The main point is this: strive to live up to your inherent structural height. Your friends may tell you that you've lost weight or simply that you look better. Only you will know that you're at your best mainly because you are filling the space to which you are entitled.

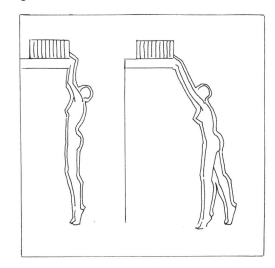

The Book of Stretches

anatomy of a stretch

In this part of your program, a special technique of stretching will help you to explore and increase the elastic capacity of your body. Elasticity is the key to good muscle tone, shapeliness, and well-coordinated graceful movement.

Muscle tone is generally judged by the size and firmness of muscles—but firmness could be a symptom of tension and size a wholly undesirable over-development. Good muscle tone is determined by the degree of elasticity, or resilience, in the muscles—that pneumatic quality of recoil, or spring, that projects vitality and animation.

The extraordinary elasticity of your muscles allows them both to stretch and to return to their original size.

When a muscle contracts, it may shorten to half its resting length. When it stretches, it may exceed its resting length up to 1½ times. But resting lengths are variable: a tense muscle will not return to its normal resting length after contracting, while a slack muscle will remain longer than normal after being stretched.

Tense or slack muscles are like ill-fitting clothes, either too tight or too loose. This accounts for the rigid, even brittle, appearance and angular movements of tense bodies, and the blurred pendulous contours of bodies that lack good muscle tone. With tensions released and natural resilience restored, muscles fit the body properly. Tense muscles become pliable and slack muscles shorten and wrap more closely around their supporting frame. Like a well-fitting girdle, they take up slack flesh and redistribute it in firmer and smoother contours.

The effectiveness of stretching increases when you balance the distribution of your efforts.

One of your primary needs is a balance of muscular power, yet the general inclination is to use larger and more familiar muscle groups for tasks that should logically be done by smaller muscle groups. Such uneven demands on the body create the imbalance of muscle tone that deprives it of good coordination. Uneven demands also invite tensions and fatigue. To develop a balance of power in your body, you must curb the tendency of your stronger muscles to dominate weaker ones.

To prevent your stronger muscles from participating at the beginning of a stretch, keep them relaxed and inhibited until you have explored the total elastic capacity of your weaker muscle groups.

Try the following example.

a) Stand upright, arms relaxed, heels together, feet slightly turned out. Assume that the muscles in the shaded area are weak and need toning.

b) Assume that the muscles in this shaded area are stronger and tend to dominate.

c) Keeping your left shoulder relaxed, support the weight of your left arm by placing your left hand on top of your head.

d) Stretch the muscles in the shaded area by bending slowly toward the right side. Explore their total elastic capacity.

e) Complete the stretch by using your right shoulder, arm, and hand freely. Relax. Resume your starting position.

If certain movements make it impossible to adjust your position in order to inhibit stronger muscle groups, rely on your muscle sense to help you balance your efforts.

The purpose of stretching is not to make muscles longer, but to increase their elasticity. To restore the resilience tense or slack muscles have lost, control the process of lengthening and shortening your muscles, and give equal value to all phases of a stretch.

To demonstrate how this works, consider a rubber band. When you stretch a rubber band, you have a number of choices. You can lengthen it either quickly or slowly; let it snap back to its original size; retain it at any length you like by controlling its power to return; or reduce its length gradually. You have the same options when you stretch your muscles—but it is the slow increase and gradual decrease of length that best restore resilience.

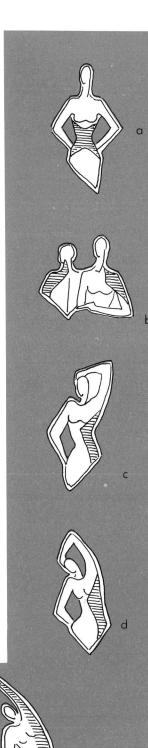

During stretches that involve your whole body, effort should originate in the center of your body, about two inches below your navel. Energy should flow from this point toward your fingertips and toes. When you reach the natural limit of a stretch, reverse the flow: relax from the extremities back to the center of your body.

In the following example, distribute your efforts evenly during the first phase of the stretch, then gradually relax and reduce its length.

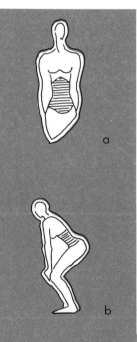

a) Stand upright, arms relaxed, heels together, feet slightly turned out. Concentrate on the area between your hips and breastbone, which has great but often unexplored elastic capacity.

b) With torso upright, arms straight, bend your knees and place your hands on them.

c) Prevent your shoulders from participating at the beginning of the stretch. Bending your arms, move your hips back as far as possible. Slide your hips from side to side, coaxing greater length from your torso.

d) Retain this length. With shoulders, arms, and hands relaxed, move your arms forward to shoulder level.

e) Do not allow your shoulders and arms to dominate the action as you continue to stretch forward from the center of your body.

f) After you have explored the total elastic capacity of your torso, stretch your shoulders, arms, and hands freely.

g) Hold your position as you allow your stretch to lessen in length and intensity. Begin by slowing relaxing your hands, arms, shoulders and upper back.

When relaxation is complete and you feel that your muscles have returned to their original length, lower your arms and resume your starting position.

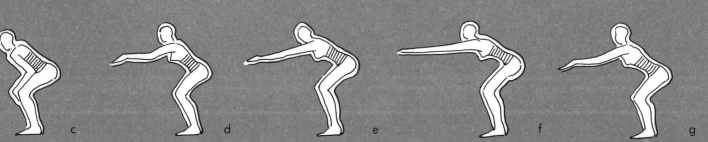

By replacing energy flow with relaxation, and without altering your position, you have relaxed above a stretch, or relaxed in position. When these phrases appear in your instructions, they will signal this process of control and gradual relaxation.

Instructions to move "smoothly," to "slide," or to "yield" indicate movements that are effortless.

The term "wrapping" describes the sensation of muscles tightening in a given direction. For example, the muscles of your thighs "wrap" diagonally upward from front to back. You can easily see and feel this directional wrapping.

As you stretch, the length of your body increases. Instead of letting it snap back to zero, like a rubber band, increase and decrease the stretch rhythmically, but plan to retain a fraction of the added length as you return to your starting position. Such a small increase requires little effort, and is instantly rewarding because an increase in torso length is always accompanied by a decrease in circumference.

Imagine a scale from 1 to 10. Let 10 stand for the length of a total stretch.

a) Stand upright, arms relaxed, heels together, feet slightly turned out. Assume that the area between your breastbone and your hips extends from 1 to 5 in resting position.

b) Raise both arms and stretch upward to increase your length to 7.

c) Relax above the stretch and lower your left arm. Bend toward the left and increase your length to 10.

d) Play the stretch like an elastic band, increasing and decreasing its length between 10 and 7. Do this 6 times.

e) Slowly lower your right arm and, as you return to starting position, retain a small portion of the length you have gained. The area that measured 5 should now measure 5½ or 6.

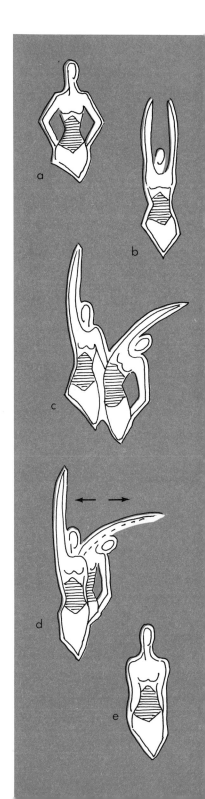

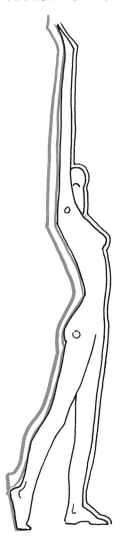

Because the following stretch sequences are designed to develop particular muscle groups, you must pay close attention to correct positioning. Your instructions suggest what reactions to feel in response to a movement. If you fail to feel an anticipated sensation, <u>adjust your position before continuing.</u> Your knees, perhaps, or your hips may have moved from their correct placement, possibly no more than an inch. A small deviation makes the difference between the success or failure of a movement.

Thinking of positioning and movements in terms of patterns will not only help you to maintain correct positions, but will also influence the quality of your movements. As you progress from Basic Stretches to Dynamic Stretches and last to the choreographed Patterned Stretches in this section, you will realize that movement is as much a means for self-expression as it is for self-development.

After you have completed the Patterned section, memorize a few of your favorite sequences. When you practice them in front of a mirror, you will discover something that I have known for many years—a body grows more beautiful by moving beautifully.

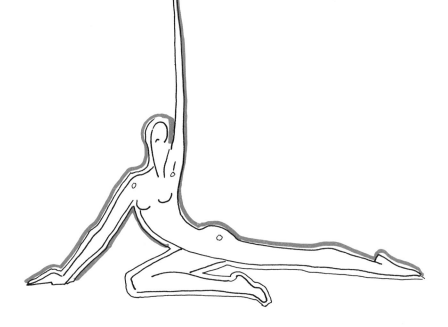

The Stretches

This part of your program consists of three sets of graded stretch sequences: 10 Basic, 10 Dynamic, and 10 Patterned Stretches (another way of saying beginning, intermediate, and advanced). To make this part of your training yield all it has to offer, move slowly enough at all times to keep your breathing normal. Your muscles need oxygen in order to work and develop. Control your energy output; use only as much energy as a movement requires and keep all muscles not directly involved in the movement relaxed. In other words, don't grimace, tense your hands and feet, or hold your breath. Concentrate on your sensations, which are your clue that you are moving correctly. Above all, relax completely after each effort.

program for basic stretches

"Once each" may mean once each, or once on each side,
or once in each direction, whichever applies.

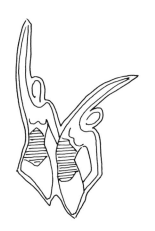

1) Practice for 3 days:

All Articulations, once each.

Posture Toning 7 to 9, once each.

Basic Stretches 1 to 4, all repeats.

2) Practice for 3 days:

All Articulations, once each.

Posture Toning 7 to 9, once each.

Basic Stretches 3 to 6, all repeats.

3) Practice for 3 days:

All Articulations, once each.

Posture Toning 7 to 9, once each.

Basic Stretches 5 to 8, all repeats.

4) Practice for 3 days:

All Articulations, once each.

Posture Toning 7 to 9, once each.

Basic Stretches 7 to 10, all repeats.

program for dynamic stretches

Continue as above, but eliminate Posture Toning 7.

program for patterned stretches

Continue as above, but eliminate Posture Toning 7 and 9.
Continue with Posture Toning 8.

Basic Stretches

1

1) Rest on your back, feet slightly apart, arms along your sides, palms up. Do not lift your chin. Bend both knees slightly, feet parallel and flat on the floor.

2) Slowly lift your left arm, keeping it straight and parallel to your body, until it is at a right angle to your body. Pressing upward from the shoulder, stretch your arm, hand, and fingers toward the ceiling. Feel the effort in your armpit and shoulder. Continuing to stretch your arm, move it slowly beyond your head and lower it to the floor. Feel the stretching sensation in the areas of the breast, armpit, and shoulder. Relax. Repeat with your right arm.
Without allowing your hips to move, raise and lower your rib cage slightly. Feel your back arching.

3) Keeping your leg bent, raise your right knee not more than 1 inch above the level of your left knee. Feel this effort in the area of your right groin.

4) Without turning your knee out, and with toes pointed, stretch your right leg until it is perfectly straight. Continue to stretch as you slowly lower your leg, stopping when it is barely above the floor. Feel a strong pull in the lower abdominal area and a contraction in the buttocks. Lower your leg to the floor. Moving from the groin, stretch your leg farther. Relax. Repeat with your left leg.

5) Gradually tighten the buttock muscles. Feel the muscles of your thighs wrapping. Holding this contraction, firmly flex your feet. Feel a strong pull in the calves and along the backs of your thighs. Relax. Slowly flex and arch your feet 3 times.

6) Press down in your calves and heels as you raise your hips from the floor. Do not lift beyond comfort. Keep your hips suspended for a slow count of 3. Feel a powerful reaction in the muscles of your back, abdomen, and legs. Lower your hips to the floor and relax.

7) Place your feet parallel and flat on the floor, bending your knees. Keeping your arms straight and parallel, raise them slowly to a vertical position, then lower them along your sides. Lift then lower your rib cage without allowing your hips to move. Relax.

Do this sequence 3 times on each side.

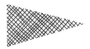

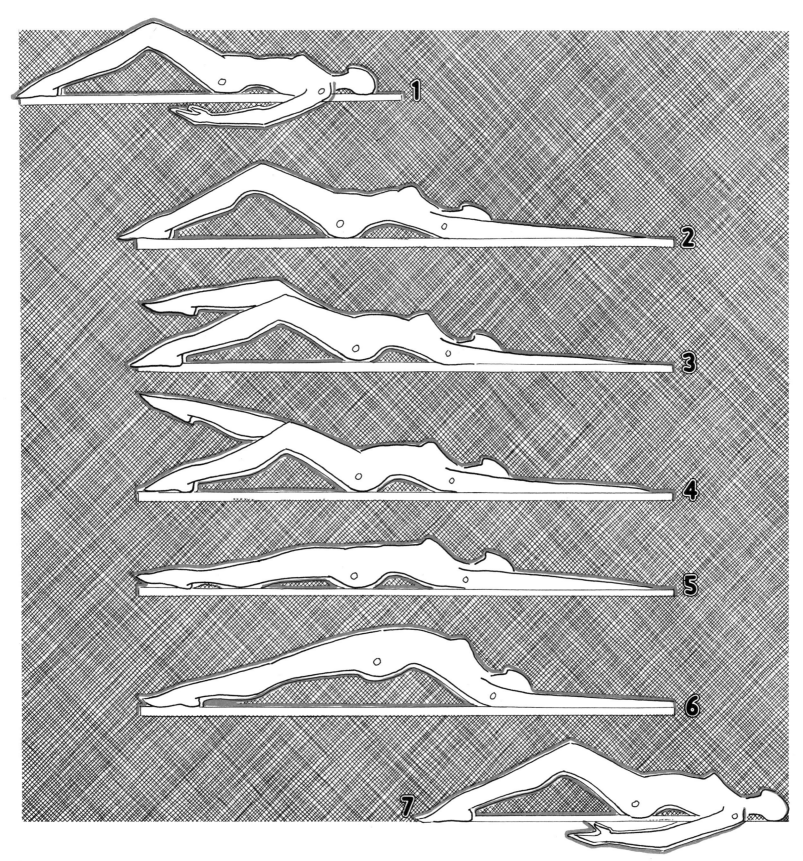

1) Rest on your back, arms on the floor beyond your head, feet together. Do not turn your knees out. Lift your rib cage slightly. Slowly and firmly flex and arch your feet 3 times. Relax. (See page 35 in Articulations on how to flex and arch.)

2) Bending your knees slightly, place your feet, heels together, flat on the floor. Keeping your head on the floor, move your arms, a shoulders' width apart, diagonally forward. Lift your shoulders and press your arms forward from the center of the armpits. Feel a strong contraction in the area of the breast, shoulders, and diaphragm.

3) Place your right foot on your left knee. Place your hands on your right knee. With face relaxed, lower your chin toward your chest and move your head forward. Keeping your left leg on the floor, move your head, shoulders, and upper back forward, allowing your arms to bend. Feel a strong contraction in the diaphragm area and lower abdomen.

4) In the same position, drop your arms, then slowly lower your head and torso to the floor. Relax. With palms down, move your arms slowly upward and beyond your head and rest them on the floor. This movement will cause your back to arch. Relax in position.

5) Lower your right leg and, with feet together, slowly straighten your legs. Do not turn your knees out. Slowly and firmly flex and arch your feet 3 times.

Do this sequence 3 times on each side.

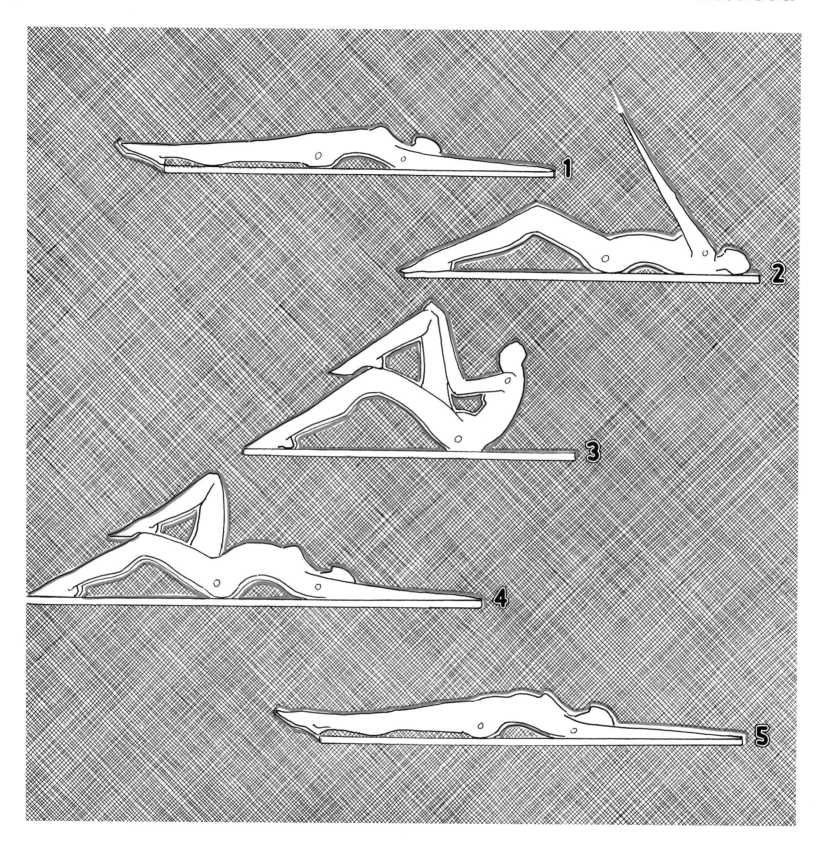

3

1) Supporting yourself on your hands and knees, your hands a shoulders' width apart, spread your fingers. With arms straight, roll the wells of your elbows forward. Feel the inner surfaces of your upper arms tightening. Rotate your head slowly in a clockwise circle, then counterclockwise. Pressing down firmly with the hands and shoulders, arch your back and lift your head and chest. Relax in position.

2) Slide your right leg back, keeping your toes on the floor. With your leg straight and the centers of your knee and instep facing the floor, press back at the back of your knee. Feel a strong pull above your kneecap and a contraction in the buttock and hip.

3) Stretch your right leg fully, keeping your chest high. Flex your right foot. Feel a contraction in your calf and buttock muscle. Relax your foot. With your right leg in position, do not lift your shoulders or allow your neck and face to tense as you lift and lengthen your torso as far as possible, without shifting your hips back.

4) Move your right leg back to the starting position. Move both hands forward by the length of one hand. With your feet relaxed and your arms completely straight, very slowly shift your hips back and lower them to your heels. Feel a strong stretching sensation along your entire back, including the area near the armpits and along the upper arms. If necessary, modify the position of your hands. Relax your neck and lower your head toward the floor. Rest, holding for a slow count of 3. Return to position 1).

Do this sequence 3 times on each side.

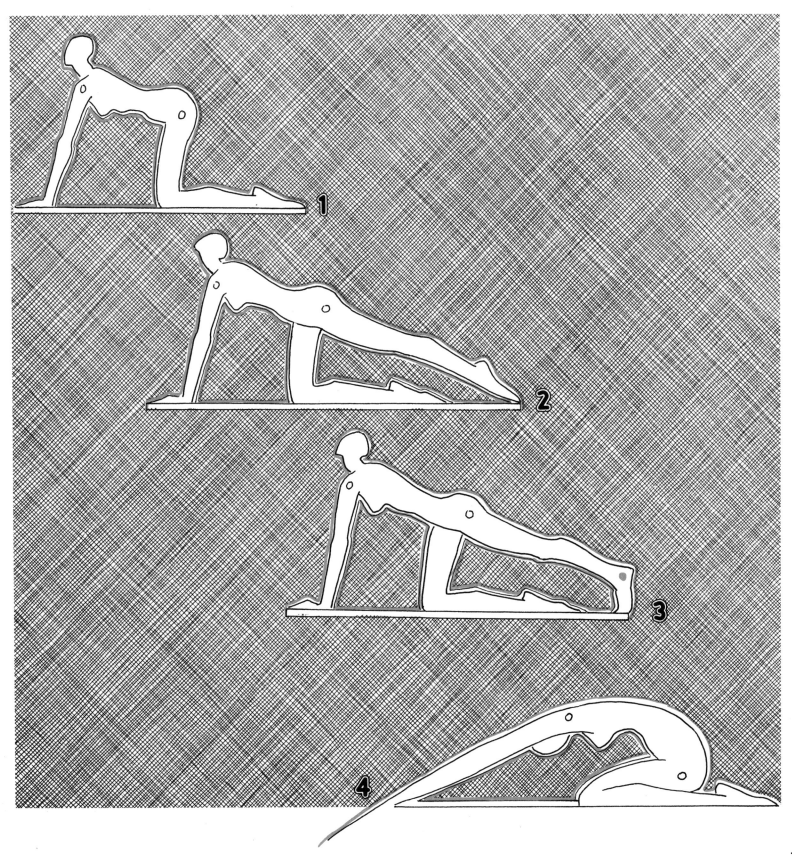

1) Sit on the floor, knees bent, feet and knees slightly separated, hands on your knees. Relax and slump. Shift from side to side on your buttocks until you feel the bony knobs of your sitting bones. Shift your torso forward until your weight rests on the center of your sitting bones, then shift forward again until it rests in front of them.
Leading with the top of your head, without lifting your chin, slowly stretch upward. Your spine will follow until your back is perfectly straight. Lower your shoulders, and lift your breastbone slightly. Move back beyond the sitting bones. Alternate between these two positions 6 times.

2) Sitting well forward on your sitting bones, without turning your knee out, straighten your left leg and bounce the knee gently up and down 6 times. Place both hands on your right knee. Straighten your left arm and move it to shoulder level. Lift and lower your left shoulder.
Holding your torso upright, and resisting the impulse to bend your left knee, move your torso gently forward and back from the hip joints 6 times. Feel a strong pull in the thigh and at the back of the left leg. Relax, drop your arms, and slump.

3) Straighten your right leg. Move forward on your sitting bones and straighten your back and legs. Do not turn your knees out. Move both arms to shoulder level; lift and lower your shoulders. With legs straight, move your torso gently forward and back from the hip joints 6 times. Feel a powerful pull along the backs of the thighs and knees. Drop your arms and gently bounce your knees up and down 6 times.

4) With your back straight, move both arms forward to slightly above shoulder level. Keep your face and neck relaxed as you slowly lean back. Feel your abdominal muscles tightening. Lifting your rib cage slightly, move your torso no farther forward than to the upright position. Feel an increased pull in your thighs. Move forward and back from the hip joints 4 times. Drop your arms and slump. Gently bounce your knees up and down 6 times. Relax.

5) With your back straight, move both arms forward and to shoulder level. Moving from the hip joints, lean your torso as far forward as possible. Feel a powerful pull in the thighs and hips. Keep your rib cage high as you return to the vertical position. Move back and forth 4 times. Drop your arms and slump. Gently bounce your knees up and down 6 times. Relax.

Do this sequence 2 times on each side.

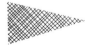

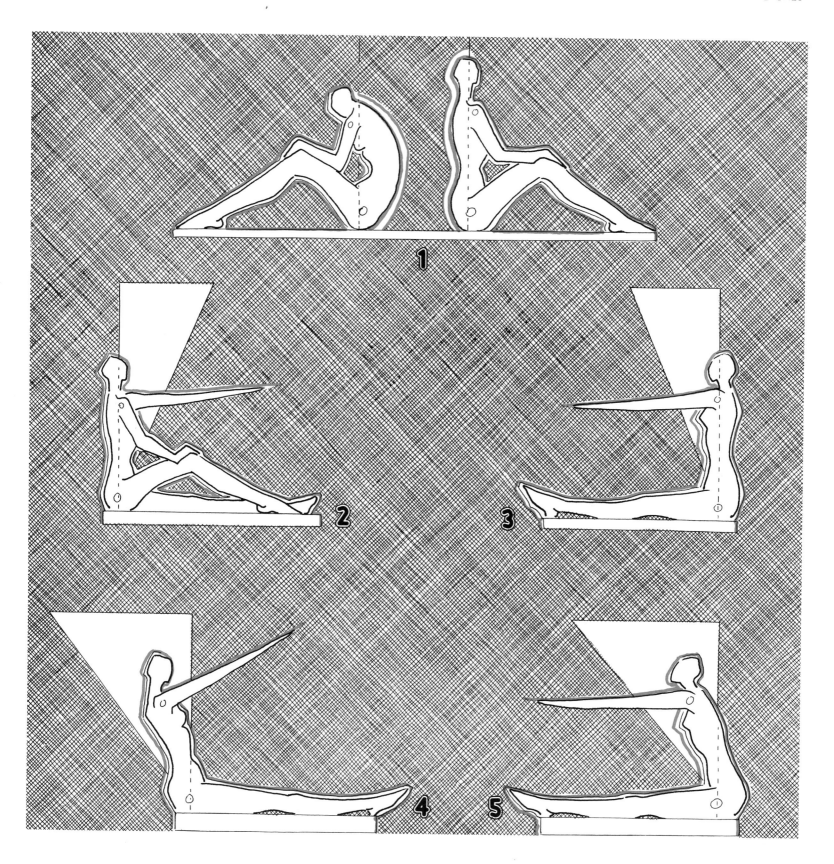

1) Sit on the floor, on your right side, knees bent, feet together. Place your left hand on your heels. Place your right palm on the floor, at a comfortable distance from your body, in line with your hips. Spread your fingers. Make sure that your shoulders face forward and that you do not slump or arch your back. Roll the well of your right elbow forward. Feel a response in the inner surface of your upper arm.

2) Press firmly down with your right hand as you lift your rib cage. Feel an increase in the length of your torso. Place your left thumb on your left shoulder.

3) Move your left arm diagonally upward until it is straight. Look up at your hand. Stretch your torso slowly upward from the groin. Without straining, stretch to full capacity. Include your hand and fingers in the stretch. Lean slightly forward and relax.

4) Lower your left arm and place your left thumb on your right shoulder. Keeping your torso high, straighten your left leg in line with the hip. Do not allow your hips to move back. Feel a powerful contraction in the buttock and in the inner surface of the thigh. If you fail to feel these sensations, move your leg back slightly and press firmly back at the knee.

5) With your leg straight, slowly raise your arm, stretching upward to full capacity. Feel the stretch permeating your entire body. With an easy motion, return to position 1) and relax.

Do this sequence 3 times on each side.

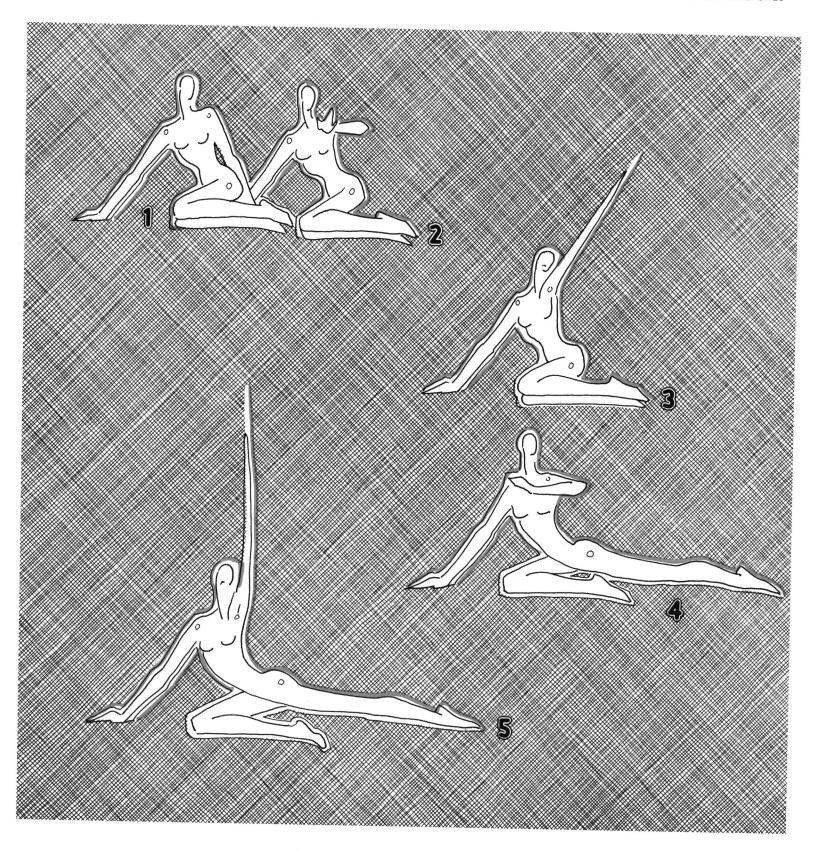

1) Stand upright, heels together and feet slightly turned out. Shift your weight to the balls of your feet, with most of your weight on the big toes and the toes next to them. Bend your knees slightly, allowing your torso to roll forward and down. Drop your head and let your arms hang loosely.

2) Without pressing excessively at the back of the knees, straighten your legs. This will cause your weight to shift back to the heels. To relieve strain at the back of the legs, shift your weight to the balls of your feet. Raise your head slightly.

3) Place your hands where your buttocks join your legs. Lift your head and torso slightly and ease your rib cage forward. Moving from the hip joints, gently lift and lower your torso 6 times. Feel your thigh muscles responding.

4) Keep your neck and face relaxed and, without straining, lift your torso only slightly upward and slide your shoulder blades together. This will cause your back to arch. Relax your shoulders. Keeping heels and toes on the floor, shift your weight toward the balls of your feet, then back to your heels, 6 times. Feel an increased pull in the leg muscles as you shift between these positions.

5) Do not lift your rib cage, but allow your spine to relax as you tilt your pelvis under and forward, keeping your knees straight. Feel a powerful wrapping sensation in the buttocks and thighs, and a strong contraction in the abdomen.

6) Drop your arms along your sides, with palms facing back. While leading upward and back with the back of your neck, shift your weight well forward to the balls of your feet. Your body will feel very light as you arrive at a fully elevated position.

7) Keeping your weight on the balls of your feet, lift and lower your toes firmly 3 times. Relax. Slowly move both arms forward and above your head. Without straining, lift your shoulders high and stretch to full capacity. Relax above the stretch, then slowly lower your arms and rest.

Do this sequence 3 times.

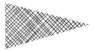

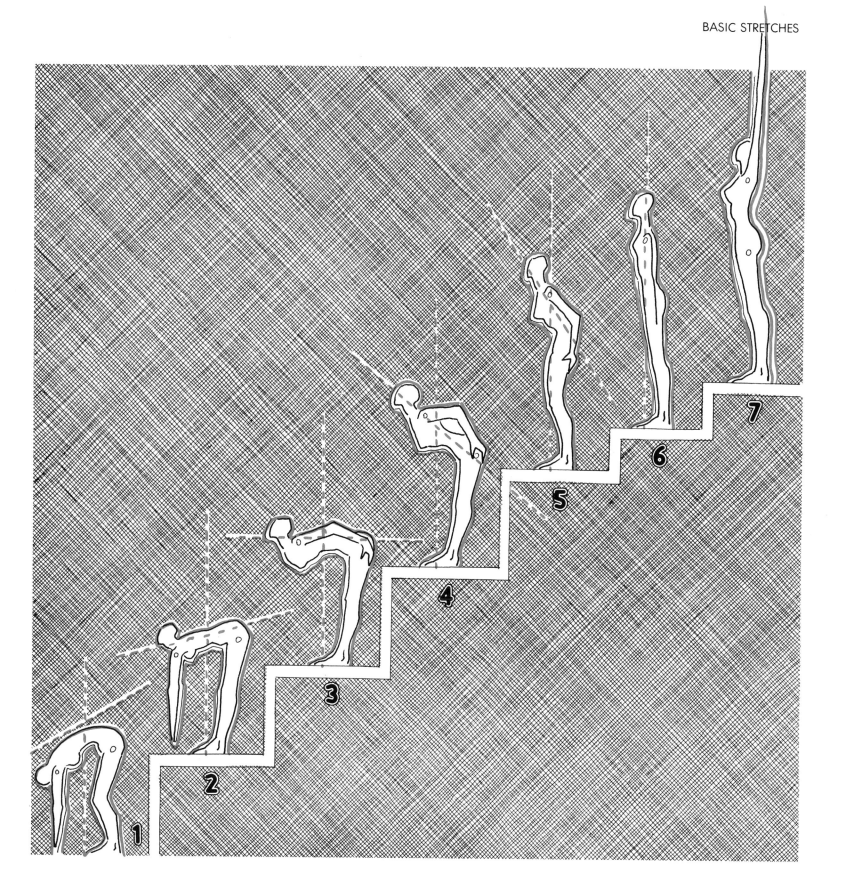

1) Stand upright, heels together and feet slightly turned out. With your weight on the balls of your feet, bend and separate your knees. Do not allow your heels to lift. Place your hands on your knees and, with shoulders low, brace your weight on your fully stretched arms. Move your hips back, arching your back as much as possible without straining. Lift your head. <u>Feel your abdomen flattening and the weight on your thighs increasing.</u> Slowly lift and lower your toes 6 times. Drop your arms and straighten your legs. Return to the upright position.

2) With your weight on the balls of your feet, bend and separate your knees, without allowing your heels to lift. Place your hands on your knees, arms straight, without bracing your weight. Ease your hips back, then move them forward, allowing your spine to curve. <u>Feel a strong reaction in the legs, buttocks, and abdomen.</u> Relax in position. Slowly return to the upright position.

3) Bend and separate your knees again and place your hands on them. Without allowing your heels to lift, deepen your knee bend. Lower your torso, bending your elbows as you move your hips back as far as possible. Relax in position and press your shoulder blades together slightly. Lengthen your torso and neck.

4) Still in position, stretch your left arm back as far as possible and place your right hand on your right shoulder. Then slowly stretch your right arm forward, including your hand in the stretch. Hold for a slow count of 3. Relax. Drop your arms and slowly return to the upright position.

Do this sequence 2 times on each side.

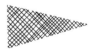

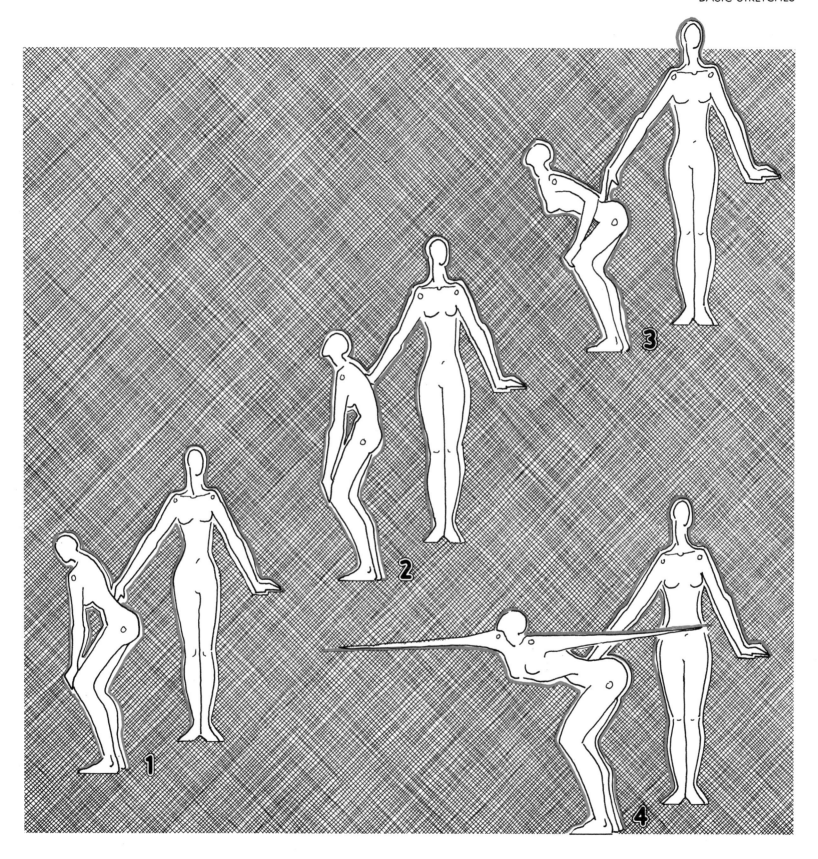

1) Stand tall, heels together and feet slightly turned out. Shift your weight forward to the balls of your feet. Move your arms slightly away from your sides.

2) Place your right arm behind your back, resting the back of your hand against your left hip. Relax. With the palm of your left hand turned out, slowly raise your left arm above your head. Stretch your entire body in the direction of the lifted arm and hold for a slow count of 3. Moving from the base of the neck, lift and lower your head 6 times. Relax.

3) Shift your weight to the balls of your feet. Relax. With your legs straight, move your left hip as far as possible to the left. Leading with the left arm, lean very slightly to the right.

   Keeping your neck, face, and your right shoulder relaxed, stretch your left arm as far as possible toward the right without straining. Inhale; exhale. Feel a strong pull along the left side of your abdomen and chest, and a compression in the right hip and waist. Relax above the stretch.

   Slowly lower your left arm as you move your left hip toward the center. Return to position 1). Rest.

   Do this sequence 3 times on each side.

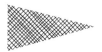

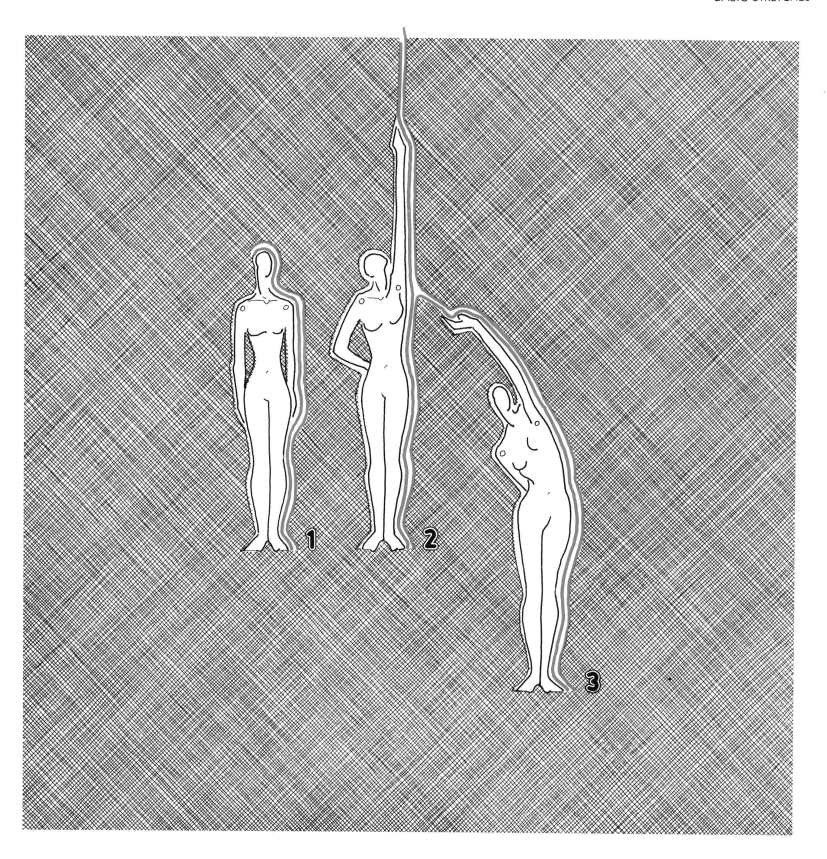

1) Stand upright with heels together, feet slightly turned out, arms relaxed. Shift your weight to the balls of your feet. Slowly move your arms forward, palms down, to just below shoulder level.

   Lift your rib cage. Slowly raise your arms above your head, and separate them slightly. Turn your hands so that your thumbs point forward and palms out, then slowly move your arms back and down, as you complete a large, circular movement. Repeat 6 times. Relax.

2) Lift your head and rib cage, and arch your back. Relax in position. Place your hands on the backs of your thighs. Open your mouth slightly and roll your head back. Relax.

   Move your shoulder blades together, then slide your hands down along your legs as far as possible. Reduce the stretch slightly and move your hands back behind your body as far as possible. <u>Feel a strong pull in your abdomen and upper arms, and across your chest.</u> Drop your arms, stand upright, and relax.

3) Bend both knees, separating them slightly. Move your hips back. Lift your shoulders as high as possible and place your hands on your knees. Lower your head to your chest.

4) Hold this position as you slowly move both arms back as far as possible without straining. Relax your arms and let them drop to your sides. Press toward the center with the inner surfaces of your upper thighs as your legs straighten. Stand tall with your weight well forward on the balls of your feet as you firmly lift and lower your shoulders 3 times. Relax.

   Do this sequence 3 times.

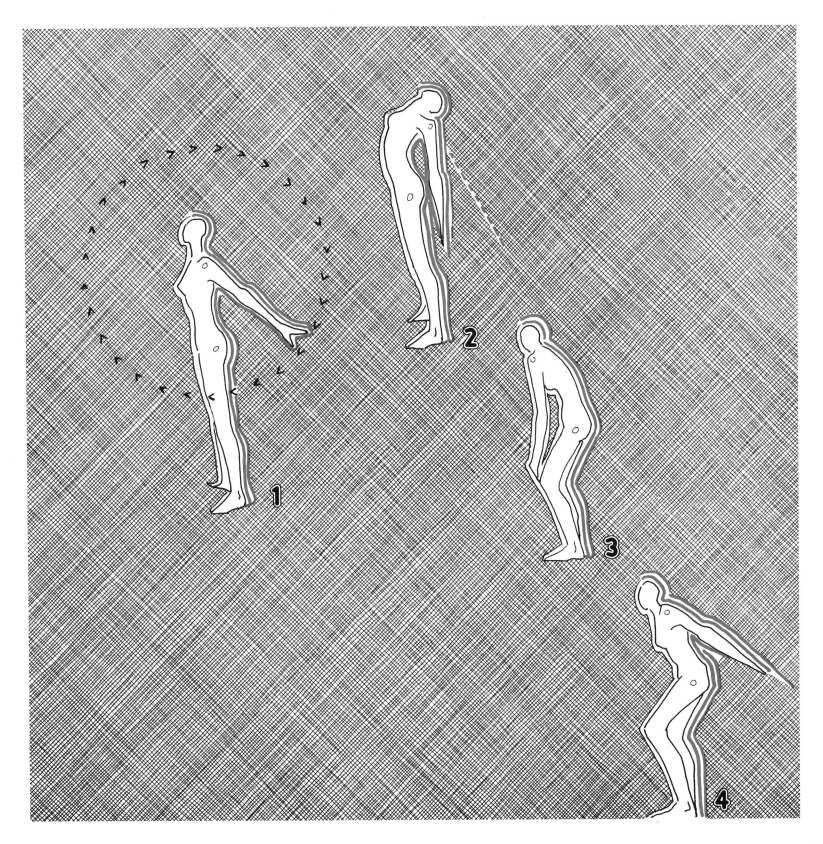

1) Sit on your right side, knees bent and feet together. Rest your right elbow on the floor in line with the back of your hips. Place your left arm behind your back. With your shoulders facing forward, raise your breastbone and lengthen the back of your neck. Move your shoulder blades together slightly. <u>Do not bear down on your elbow; your weight should rest mainly on your right thigh.</u>

2) Place your left thumb on your left shoulder. Starting at the groin, slowly stretch your torso to full capacity. Relax.

3) Move your left arm gradually upward as you straighten your left leg in line with your hip. Press firmly back at the knee. <u>Feel a strong reaction in the hip, buttock, thigh, and torso.</u> Relax.

4) Slowly move your left hand and your head toward the right, allowing your body to follow. Stretch toward the right. <u>Feel a strong pull along your entire body, from ankle to hand.</u> Relax above the stretch. Lift your left leg and torso simultaneously, as you return to position 1). Relax.

Do this sequence 3 times on each side.

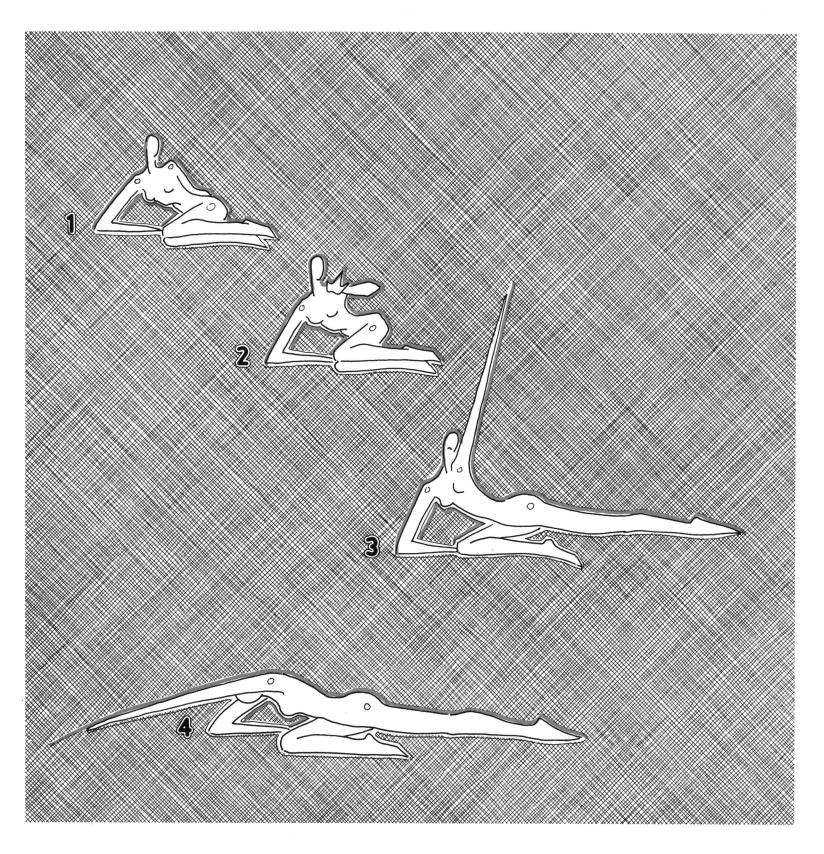

Dynamic Stretches

1) Stand upright, heels together, feet slightly turned out, arms relaxed. Shift your weight forward to the balls of your feet. Keep your heels on the floor as you bend and separate your knees. With arms straight, place your hands on your knees and lift your torso.

2) Keep your right hand on your right knee, and place your left thumb against your left shoulder, palm facing forward.

3) Move your left arm back, straightening your legs at the same time. Coax your left arm upward as far as possible. This movement will cause you to lean forward. Feel a strong pull along the hips, buttocks, and backs of your legs, and a stretching sensation in the area of your left breast, shoulder, and arm. Lower your left arm, bend your knees, then straighten your legs. Relax.

Do this sequence 2 times.

Repeat the above sequence in the following variations:
1) Place your hands midway between your ankles and knees in position 1).
2) Place your hands on your ankles in position 1). If this positioning is difficult, raise your heels and bend slightly forward.

Do these variations 2 times on each side.

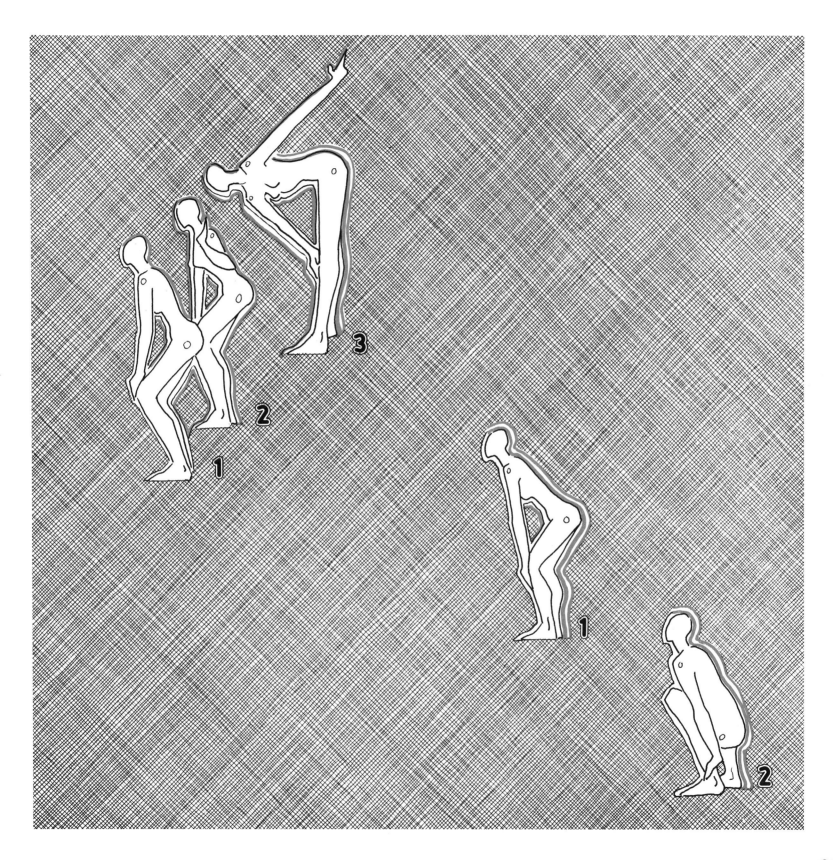

2

1) Sit on your right side, knees bent, feet together. Place your right elbow on the floor, in line with the back of your hips. Move your left arm behind your back and lift your rib cage slightly.

2) Place your left hand on your left shoulder.

3) Move your arm slowly upward until it is straight but not stiff. Look at your hand. Straighten your left leg in line with your hip, press your knee back firmly. Feel a strong contraction in the buttock and thigh. If you fail to feel this reaction, move your leg back slightly. Stretch your arm and leg thoroughly until your abdominal area feels taut. Relax above the stretch.

4) Turn your head and torso toward the right as far as comfort will allow. Shift your weight forward, stretch your left arm toward the right, then stretch your left leg, knee straight, to full capacity. Feel this stretch from your left foot, all along your body, to your left hand. Increase and decrease the length of the stretch in small to-and-fro movements, 6 times.

5) Lean slightly forward, placing your left hand on the floor. Keeping your left leg straight, raise it slightly, then move it back moderately. Lift your torso. Move your left arm slowly to the left, turning your shoulders until they face front. Turn your head to the left as you bend your left leg. Arch your back firmly, raising your rib cage, as your left hand slowly reaches for your left ankle. Feel a strong pull along the front of your body, a slight pinching at the waist, and a powerful pull along the front of your left thigh. Return to position 1).

Do this sequence 3 times on each side.

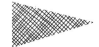

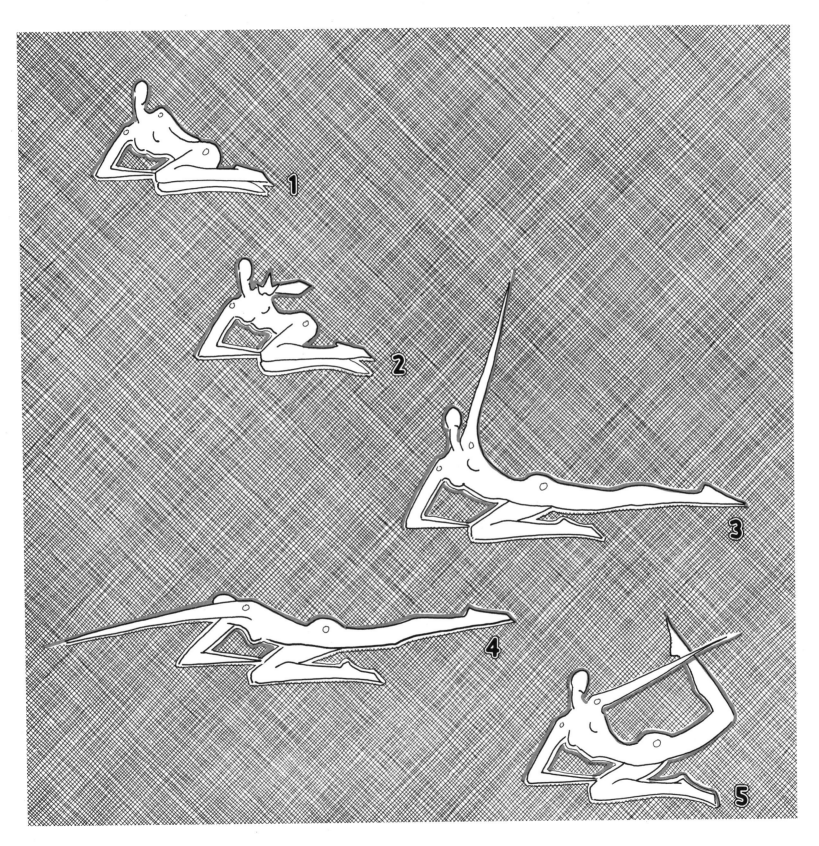

3

1) Sit on your right side, knees bent, feet together. Place your right elbow on the floor in line with the back of your hips. Move your left arm behind your back and lift your rib cage. Press your shoulder blades together firmly and relax them—3 times. Roll your left shoulder from front to back 3 times. Arch and relax your spine 3 times.

2) Place your left thumb on your left shoulder.

3) Stretch your arm up slowly until it is straight but not stiff. Look up at your hand. Straighten your left leg in line with your hip and press firmly back with your knee. Keep your hip from moving as you slowly inch your left foot backward along the floor, as far as comfort will allow. Feel a powerful contraction in the buttock and a strong pull in the inner thigh.

4) Move your right shoulder back, allowing your torso to turn toward the right. Your left arm will be stretched toward the right as you lower it to shoulder level. Stretch to full capacity. Feel the stretch from foot to hand. Relax.

5) Lift your torso and put your left thumb on your left shoulder. Place your left knee on top of your right knee. Move your right hand, palm up, closer to your right thigh. With thumb on shoulder, shift forward, twisting until your left elbow rests in your right palm, and with this motion lift and lower your torso 6 times. Feel a strong response in the twisting muscles of your waist, hip, abdomen, and upper back. Relax. Return to starting position.

Do this sequence 3 times on each side.

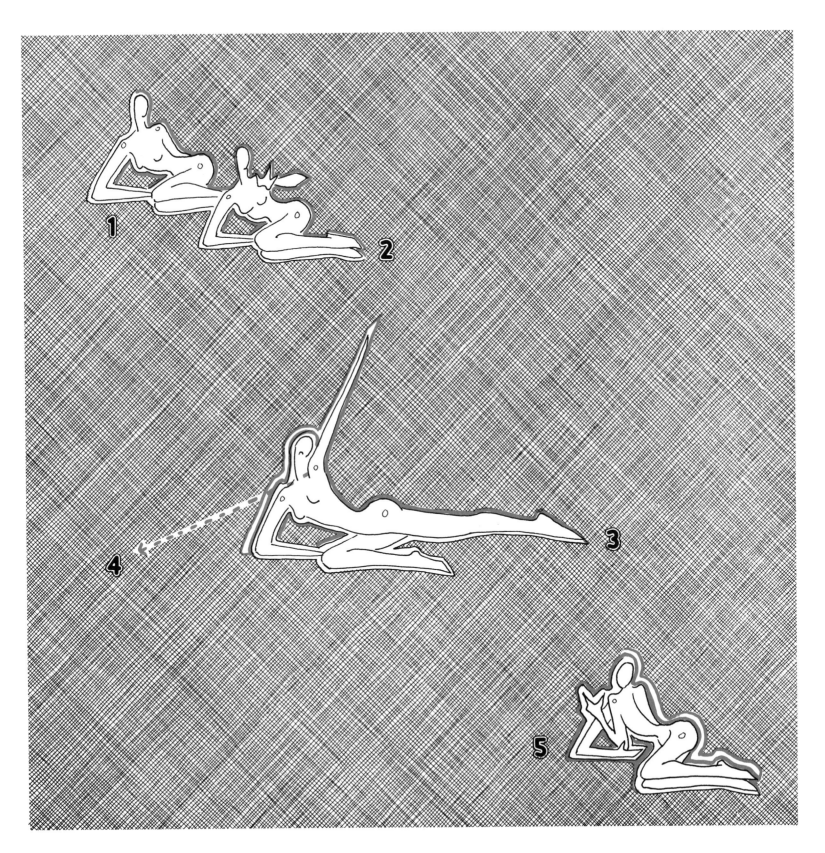

1) Rest on your back, legs slightly apart, arms along your sides. Do not allow your knees to turn out. Feel the length and weight of your body. Relax your ankles. Slowly slide your heels forward until your feet are fully flexed. Feel a strong pull in the calves. Relax. Flex and relax your feet again. With face relaxed, press your hands into tight fists, then relax them gradually.
Without tensing your toes or bending your knees, slowly arch your feet. Increase the arch by reaching toward the floor with your toes. Arch, point, and relax your feet 3 more times.

2) With your right leg straight, move your left knee slowly toward your chest. Bend and lift both elbows slightly; relax your hands and wrists. Inhale and exhale. Without pressing, lower your chin toward your chest. Lift your head and shoulders, moving them forward until your knee and elbows meet. Feel a strong reaction in the area of your diaphragm.

Relax in this position. Flex and arch your feet 3 times. With your chin close to your chest, slowly lower your head and shoulders to the floor. Lower and relax your arms.

3) Slowly stretch both arms and your left leg upward until they are straight and at right angles to your body. If the straightening of your leg at this angle is beyond your present capacity, raise it somewhat less. Relax in this position. Gently flex and arch your feet 3 times.

4) Stretch your arms and your left leg in opposite directions, as you gradually lower them to the floor. Feel a powerful pull in the abdomen, a strong response in the breasts, chest, and upper arms. Relax.

5) Inhale and exhale deeply. Starting at the groin, slowly contract your abdomen. Holding the contraction, firmly flex and arch your feet 3 times. Inhale and exhale deeply. Return your arms along your sides. Rest.

Do this sequence 2 times on each side.

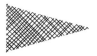

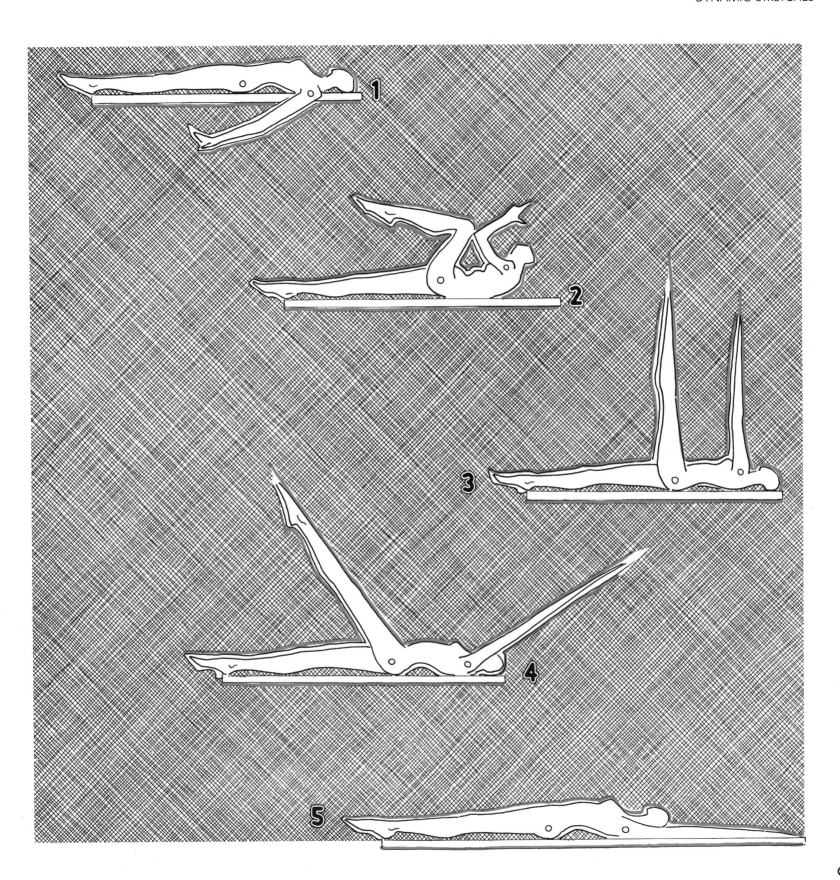

1) Sit on the floor, knees wide apart and bent, feet slightly turned out and firmly in contact with the floor, hands on knees, arms relaxed. Lean forward until you are in a "jackknife" position, <u>your weight well forward on your buttocks</u>. Slowly straighten your back and neck, and ease your shoulders. Straighten your right leg without allowing it to turn out. Bounce your knee gently up and down 6 times. Rest your left elbow on your left knee, your right hand on your right knee.

2) Lift your torso and press your right arm completely straight. <u>Feel a strong pull in the muscles of your right thigh</u>. Bounce your right knee 6 times to ease the strain, ending with the leg straight. Make a conscious effort to relax the hip muscles and place your right hand, palm facing forward, on your right shoulder.

3) Press down firmly with your left elbow and slowly move your right arm upward until it is straight. <u>Remain firmly seated</u> as you stretch to full capacity. Look up at your hand. Relax above the stretch.

4) Bend and lower your right arm to shoulder level, and turn your torso slightly to the right. Place your left hand on your right knee. With back straight, move your torso gently forward from your hip joints until your hand touches your foot. Advance and retreat in small movements 6 times. <u>Hand and foot contact is of secondary importance; the movement is designed to free the hip joints.</u>

5) Keeping your left arm completely straight, wrap your right hand around your left elbow. Relax your right foot. In this position, raise both arms forward to shoulder level, and lift your rib cage.

6) Keep your right hip firmly on the floor as you raise your arms in an easy fluid sweep above your head. Stretch upward from the rib cage and armpits. <u>Feel a strong pull in your torso and legs</u>. Lower your arms and resume position 1.

Do this sequence 3 times on each side.

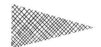

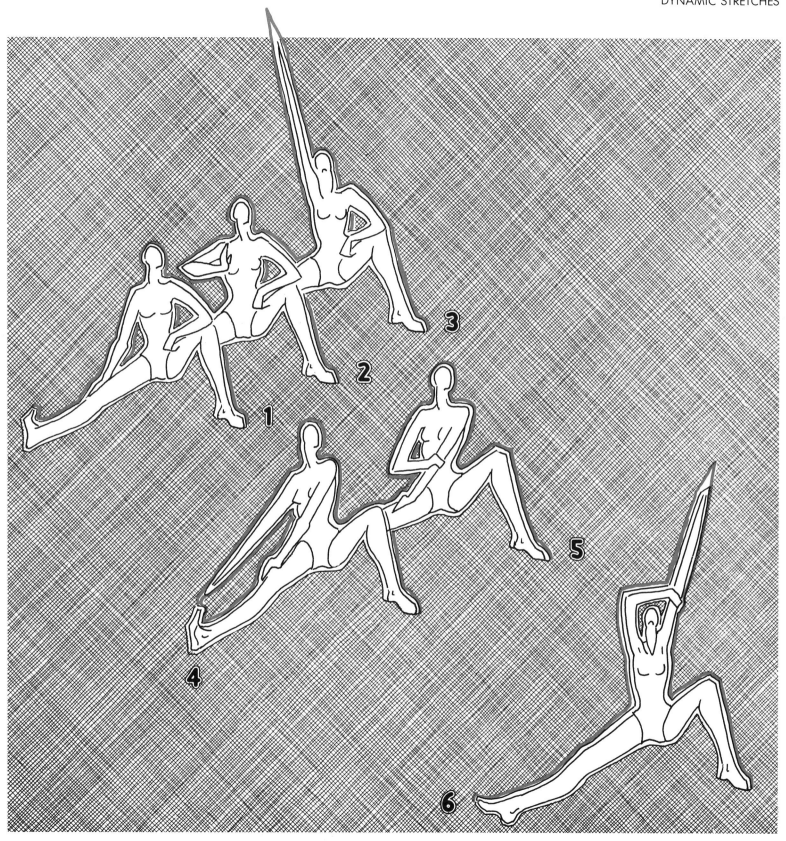

1) Rest on your stomach, arms straight ahead. Separate your legs slightly. Relax your feet and rest your legs on the <u>exact centers of your kneecaps</u>. Spread your fingers and press firmly down into your palms as you lift your head, shoulders, and chest gently upward. <u>Do not strain</u>.

2) Keep your back relaxed as you raise your head and rib cage higher. Inhale and exhale deeply. <u>Feel a strong stretching sensation along the front of your body and a contraction in the muscles of your back and buttocks.</u>

3) Keeping your hips firmly on the floor and your right arm perfectly straight, shift your weight increasingly into your left hand. Press down firmly with your left palm, as you lift your right arm to shoulder level. Without straining, stretch forward as far as possible, keeping your right arm straight. Lower your right arm. Relax.

4) With your weight still on your left hand, move your right arm and shoulders slowly to the right. Turn your head to the right as you bend your right leg. Arch your back by lifting your rib cage as high as possible, and slowly reach for your right ankle with your right hand. <u>Feel a strong contraction in the muscles of your back, hips, and buttocks, and a powerful stretching sensation along the entire front of your body.</u>

5) Move your right arm and shoulders to the front as you lower your right leg. Place your right hand on the floor; arch your back by raising your rib cage. Inhale and exhale deeply. Relax.

6) Very slowly lower your chest, shoulders, and head toward the floor, and gently lift and lower your shoulders 3 times.

Do this sequence 3 times on each side, alternating sides.

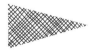

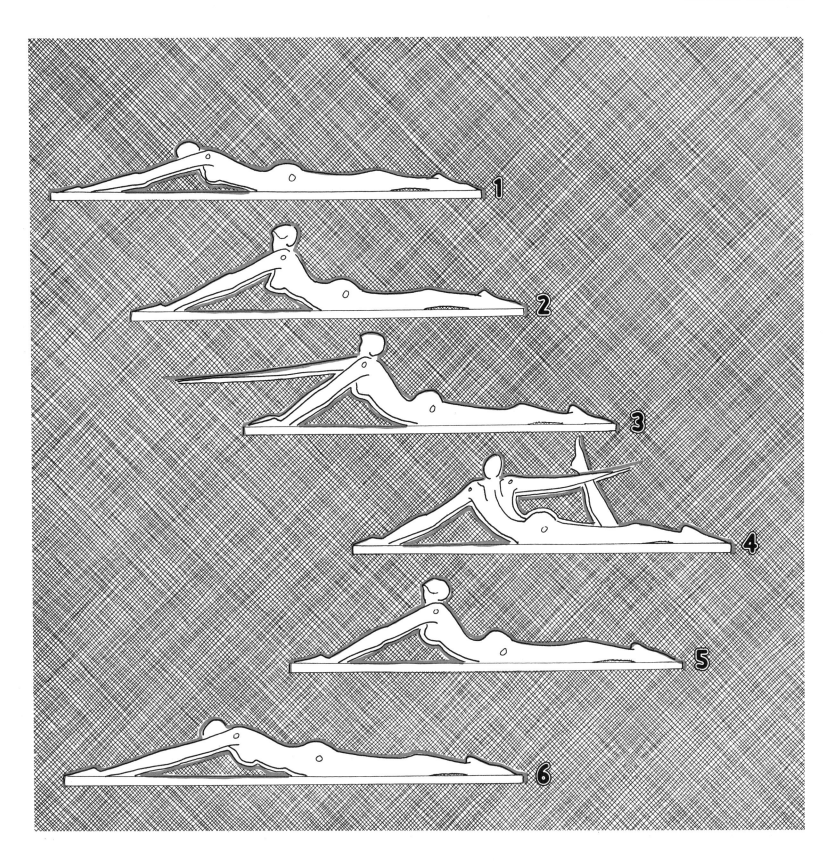

1) Sit on your right side, <u>knees sharply bent and close to your chest</u>. Place your right palm on the floor, diagonally back from your hip at a distance that will permit you to hold your torso upright. With the knee bent, lift your left leg and place it behind your hip on the floor, so that your left knee touches your right foot. This will cause your left hip to lift. Place your left hand on your right knee.

2) Shift your weight forward slightly. Spread the fingers of your right hand and roll the well of your elbow forward. <u>Feel a response in the inner surface of your upper arm</u>. Press your left hand firmly down on your right knee and stretch your torso. Relax in position. Place your left thumb on your left shoulder and turn your head toward the left.

3) Keeping your head to the left, turn your torso to the right as you stretch your left arm to the right until it is straight. This will increase the arch of your back and cause your left hip to lift higher. <u>Feel a strong reaction in the left groin and thigh, the entire abdominal area, and a strong contraction at your waist, hip, and buttock</u>. Lift and lower your left shoulder 3 times. Relax.

4) Place your left hand behind your head. Lift your rib cage.

5) Slowly move your left arm diagonally upward until it is straight. Stretch to full capacity. <u>Feel a strong contraction at your waist and hip, and a strong pull along the front of your torso.</u> Relax above the stretch.

6) While in the arched position, turn your head to the left, over your shoulder, until you see your left foot. Then move your left arm slowly down until your hand comes to rest on your left ankle. Relax, and return smoothly to position 1.

                    Do this sequence 3 times on each side.

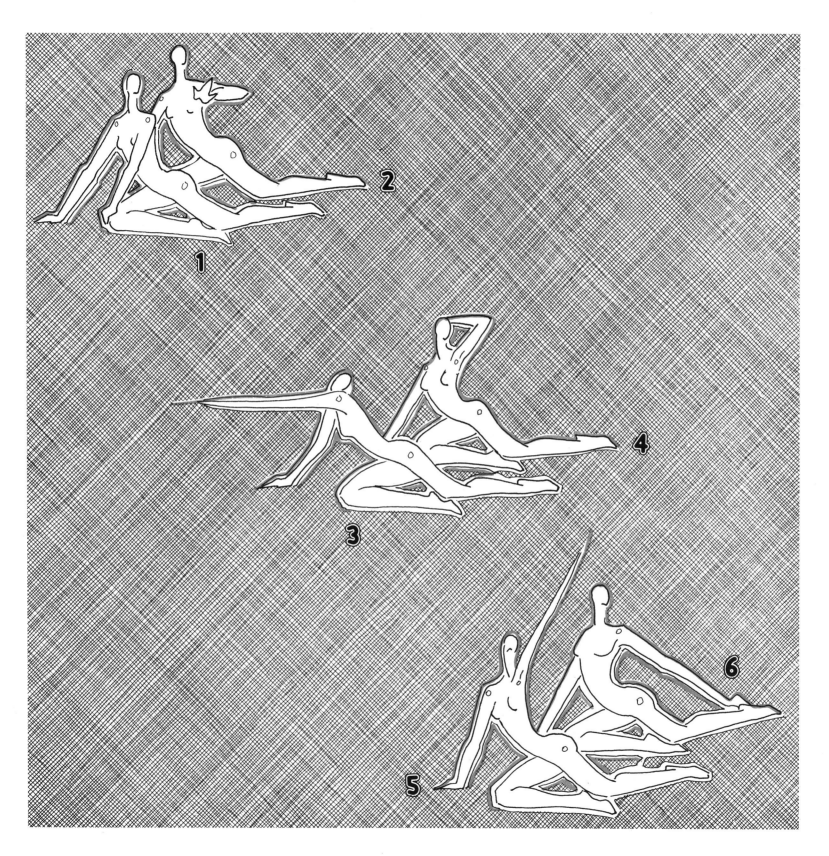

1) Stand upright, with feet apart and slightly turned out, arms relaxed. Shift your weight to the balls of your feet and avoid the tendency to settle your weight on your heels. Lengthen the back of your neck.

2) With palms down, firmly press your arms to the sides until they are at shoulder level. Keep your shoulders low. With your knees straight and without allowing your pelvis to tilt back, slowly move your left hip as far to the left as possible. Distribute your weight evenly on both feet. Relax in position.

3) Slowly raise your right arm, palm down, until it is in a diagonal line with your left hip.

4) With the same steady pressure, slowly raise your left arm until it is close to your head, and move your right arm higher. Feel a powerful pull across your torso and both arms. Relax above the stretch.

5) Shift your weight well forward to the balls of your feet. Lift your rib cage high as you move your left hip to center. Palm down, slowly press your left arm down as you stretch upward with your right arm. Maintain a feeling of rising in your torso as you slowly press your right arm down. Relax.

Do this sequence 3 times on each side.

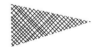

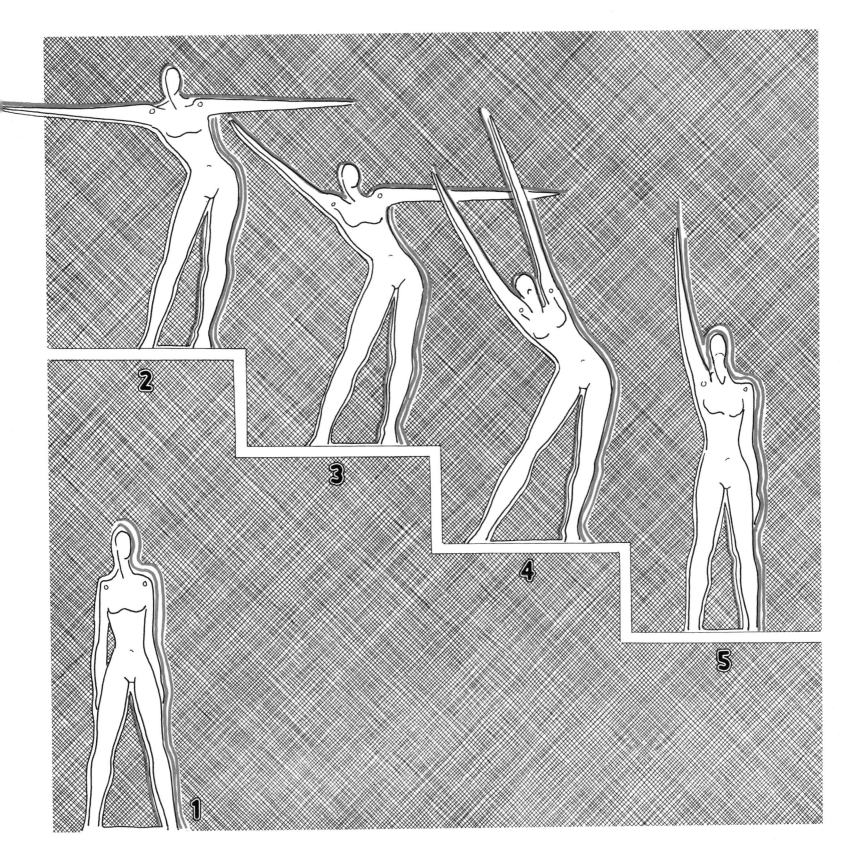

1) Stand tall, with your left side near a wall, heels together, feet slightly turned out. With your left elbow bent, place your left palm against the wall at shoulder level. Turn your right palm out and slowly move your arm sideways to above your head. Relax. Keep your arm and shoulder still. With knees straight, move your hips toward the right until your body is curved enough to allow your right hand to touch the wall without straining.

2) Place your fingers securely on the wall and stretch slowly upward. Move your fingers higher on the wall as you lengthen your body. Relax above the stretch. Press your weight down on your toes and raise your heels until you are standing securely on your toe platforms. Press your knees back firmly. Move your fingers up along the wall until the stretch is complete.

3) Keep your fingers in position on the wall. Keep your heels together as you slowly bend and separate your knees. Feel a powerful stretch all along your body.

4) Remain on your toes and keep your hips steady as you slowly straighten your knees. Feel your thighs wrapping and your buttock muscles tightening.

5) Allowing your fingers to slide down, slowly lower your heels to the floor without allowing your weight to rest on them. Lower your right arm, palm down. Relax.

Do this sequence 2 times on each side.

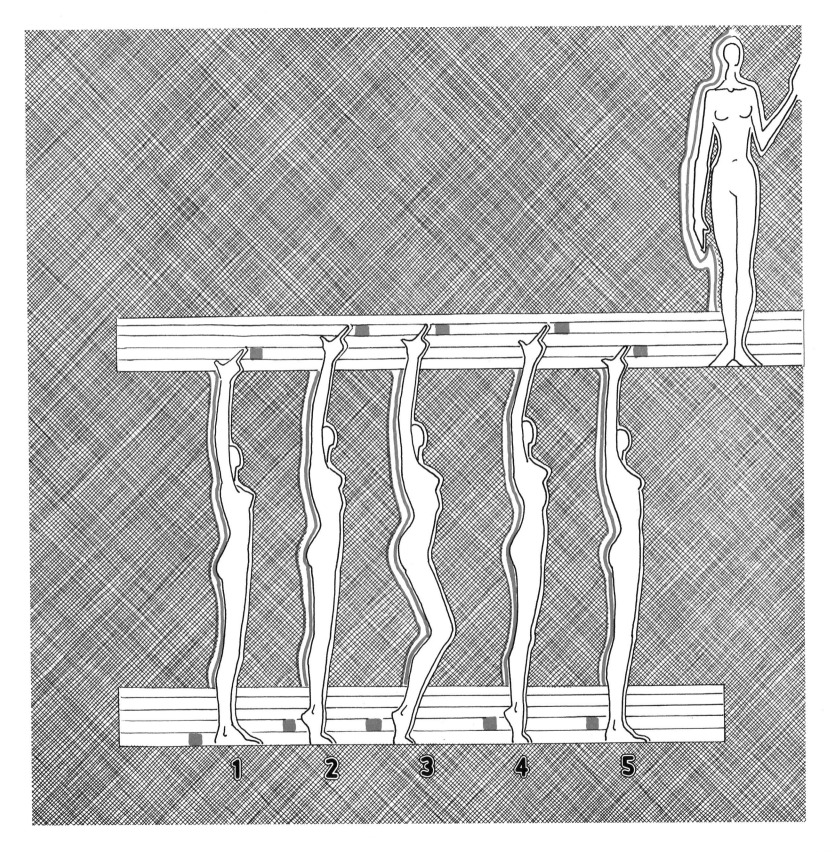

1) Stand upright, heels together, feet slightly turned out, with your left side near a wall. With left elbow bent, place your left palm against the wall at shoulder level. Relax.

Press your weight firmly into the ball of your left foot. Move your right leg straight back, <u>making sure that your right hip remains facing front</u>. Straighten your right leg, pressing the knee back. Lift your right heel, bracing your weight on the toes. Do not turn your ankle out. <u>Feel a strong contraction in the right buttock and thigh.</u>

Turn your right palm up and slowly raise your arm sideways above your head. <u>Keep both shoulders facing straight forward</u>. Stretch to full capacity. Relax above the stretch.

2) Without lowering the knee, bend your right leg at a sharp angle. Hold your torso fully upright as you lift your right leg back and upward from the hip. Allow your left knee to bend. <u>Feel a pinching sensation at your waist and hip.</u> Keep the leg elevated as you increase the arching of your back by lifting the rib cage. Slowly turn your right shoulder to the right and lower your right arm until your hand reaches your right ankle. Relax your right arm, lower your leg. Straighten both legs, and stand with feet together.

3) Bend your left leg slightly as you move your right knee forward. Keeping your torso fully erect, raise your right knee as high as possible. Hold this position as you increase the arch of your back by lifting the rib cage. Slowly turn your right shoulder to the right and stretch your arm back as far as comfort will allow. Relax. Lower your right arm and your right leg. Straighten both legs. Stand upright with feet together. Relax.

Do this sequence 3 times on each side, alternating sides.

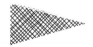

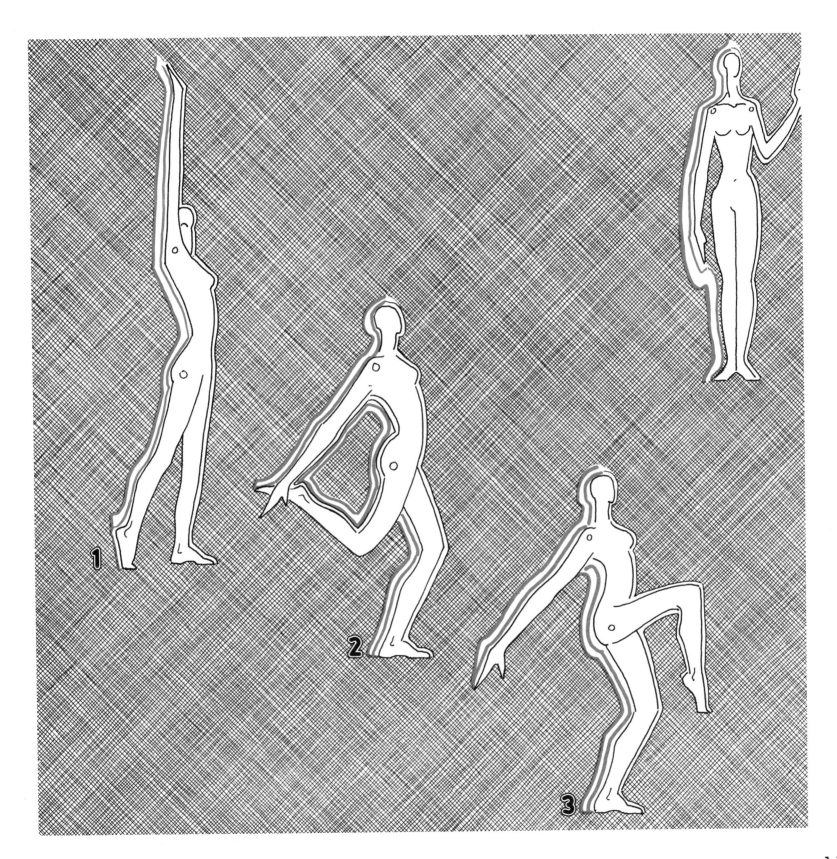

Patterned

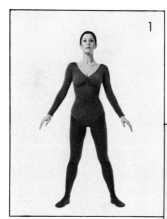

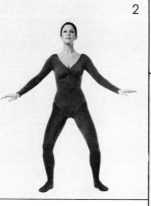

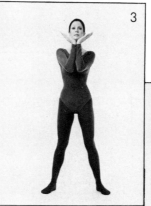

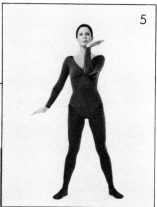

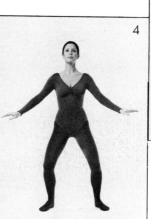

1) Stand upright, feet apart and slightly turned out, arms relaxed and slightly away from your sides. Shift your weight to the balls of your feet. Keep your shoulders low. Lift your rib cage slightly.

2) Raise your arms smoothly to just below shoulder level. Keep your torso upright as you move your hips back and bend your knees. Do not allow your heels to lift.

3) <u>Plan to press simultaneously with your elbows and your upper thighs.</u> Do not let your pelvis tilt back. Keep shoulders low. Bend your arms, press your elbows together, and simultaneously press gently inward along the inner surfaces of your upper thighs as you straighten your legs. <u>Feel a strong pull across your upper back and abdomen, a wrapping sensation in the thighs and buttocks.</u> Hold for a slow count of 3. Relax.

4) Move your arms smoothly to the sides. Keep your shoulders low. Bend your knees, moving your hips back and keeping your weight well forward on the balls of the feet. Do not allow your heels to lift. Raise your rib cage slightly; relax your neck and shoulders.

5) Place the heel of your left hand against your chin. Keep your right arm straight. Press your left elbow toward the center of your chest as you straighten your legs, pressing inward in the inner surfaces of your upper thighs. <u>Feel a pull across your upper back and at the buttocks, thighs, and abdomen.</u> Hold for a slow count of 3. Relax.

Stretches

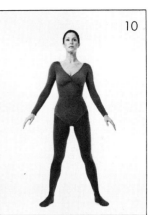

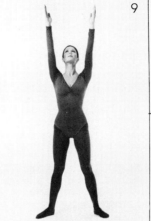

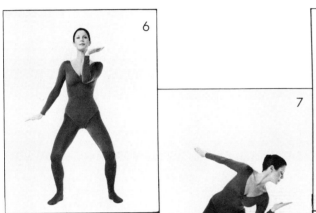

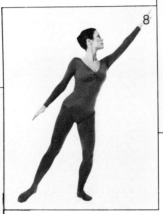

8) Keep your left knee slightly bent. Move your pelvis slightly forward. Lift your torso, raising your left arm up and to the left. Shift your weight gradually to your left leg. Stretch up and to the left until your right leg is straight. Brace your weight on the toes of your right foot. Press firmly down on both feet for balance. Lower your right shoulder and lift your rib cage. Feel a powerful stretch over your whole body.

6) Bend your knees and move your pelvis back. Move your left hand forward slightly.

7) Move your hips back as far as possible while lowering your torso until your left elbow touches your left knee. Rotate your right hand so that the palm is turned out and the thumb points back. Move your right arm back and up as far as possible without forcing. Feel a powerful pull in the hips, along your back and your right arm.

9) Shift your weight toward your right leg as you straighten your left leg. Evenly supported on both feet, shift your weight to the balls of your feet. Keep your left arm high. Relax your neck and shoulders as you raise your right arm. With chin lifted and both arms above your head, slowly stretch upward from the groin to full capacity. Relax above the stretch.

10) With palms down, slowly lower your arms. Inhale and exhale deeply 3 times. Relax.

Do this sequence 3 times on each side.

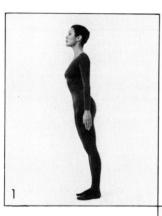

5) Continue to move your pelvis forward, drop your arms, and straighten your legs. Lift your rib cage and arch your back without straining. Roll your head back, then press your shoulders back. <u>Feel a strong pull from the center of the breasts toward the shoulders</u>. Move your arms away from the hips, increasing the arch of your back. Relax in position.

3) With arms straight, place your hands on your knees. Arch your back and move your hips back. Raise your head. <u>Feel a contraction along your back, lower abdomen, buttocks, and thighs</u>. Relax.

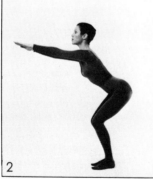
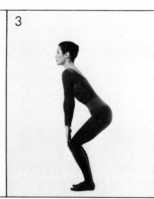
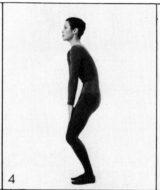
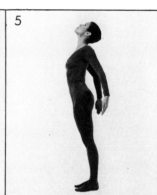

1) Stand upright, heels together, feet slightly turned out, arms relaxed. With your weight on the balls of your feet, heels on the floor, press your arms down firmly as you lengthen your spine.

2) Move both arms forward and your hips back as far as possible, while bending your knees. Stretch your back, without lifting your shoulders. <u>Feel your waist lengthening</u>. Do not pull your stomach in; it will flatten as you stretch.

4) With your weight on the balls of your feet, allow your spine to yield as you gently tilt your pelvis under and forward. <u>Feel a contraction in the buttocks, hips, abdomen, and thighs</u>. Relax.

2

6) Place your right thumb on your right shoulder. Relax your left arm. Lifting your rib cage, slowly raise your right arm upward. Press lightly downward with the left arm near the back of the legs. Shift your weight to the balls of your feet. Stretch to full capacity and relax in position. Feel a strong pull along the length of your body.

8) Lift your head slightly and, without pressing back at the knees, straighten both legs, one leg at a time. Ease any discomfort in the back of the legs by shifting your weight to the balls of your feet, and by lifting your torso slightly.

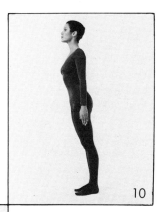

10

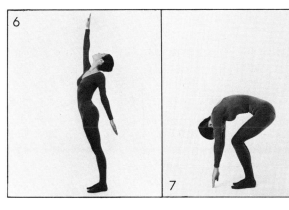

6

7

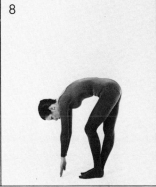

8

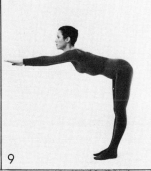

9

Lower your arms. Moving 10)
your pelvis forward slightly, lead upward with the back of the neck. Resume your starting position. Relax.

Do this sequence
2 times on each side.

7) Lower your right arm. Lower your head and torso, bend your knees, and drop your arms so your fingers touch the floor. Rest in position for a slow count of 6.

9) Move your arms, straight but not stiff, forward to shoulder level. Raise your torso to slightly above a right angle to your legs. Lengthen your torso without lifting your shoulders. Feel your abdomen flattening. Lower your chin toward your chest.

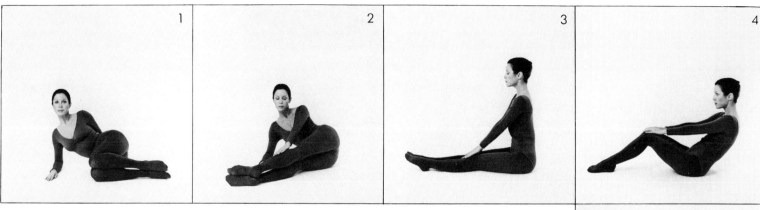

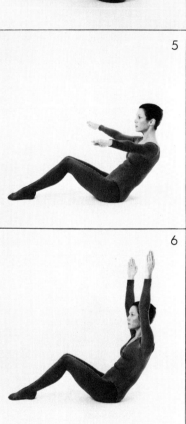

1) Rest on your right side, your elbow in line with your hips. Bend your knees and move them close to your chest. Place your left arm behind your back. Slide your shoulder blades together slightly to lift the torso.

2) In an easy sweep, straighten your legs in the direction of your supporting arm. Relax your knees and straighten your legs. Feel a pull along the back of your legs.

3) Roll over until you are in a sitting position with your weight well on the front of your buttocks and your back straight. Place your hands on your knees, then lift and lower your shoulders 3 times. Relax in position.

4) Slide your feet toward you by bending your knees. Roll back on your buttocks. Keep your arms straight, hands on knees, and relax. Adjust your neck for comfort, and relax your abdomen.

5) Hold this position, with abdomen relaxed; contractions in the abdominal wall will result from arm movements. With shoulders low, slowly lift your arms, palms down, to shoulder level. Move your arms to the sides very slowly until you feel your lower abdominal muscles tightening and pushing forward. Stop.

6) Turn your palms up, and slowly lift your arms. Keep your neck and face relaxed. Feel your abdomen flattening. As you continue to lift your arms, contractions will spread upward until the entire front of your body is taut. Hold for a slow count of 3.

3

7) With your arms above your head, ride forward on the buttocks and lift your rib cage. Sit at a right angle to the floor. Lower your arms slowly and firmly lift and lower your shoulders 3 times.

8) Lower your torso, allow your head to roll forward, place your hands on your ankles. Rest for a slow count of 6.

9) Place your hands on the floor behind your back, with fingers pointing back. Shift your weight toward your hands. Keep your body slack. Lower your head. Relax.

10) Move forward on the buttocks, lift your rib cage, and arch your back. Relax in position and let your head roll back. Feel a strong pull in the lower back, abdomen, and chest. Relax. Lift your head and straighten your back.

11) Lean slightly forward as you return to your starting position. Relax.

Do this sequence 2 times on each side.

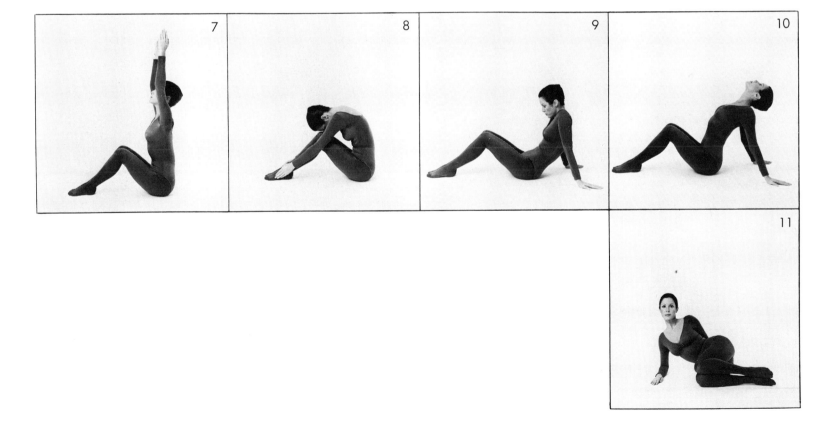

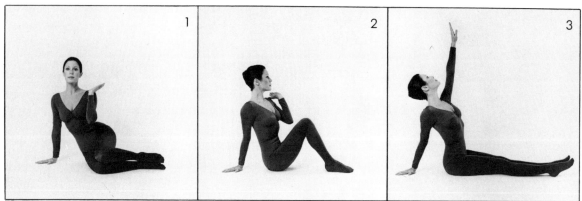

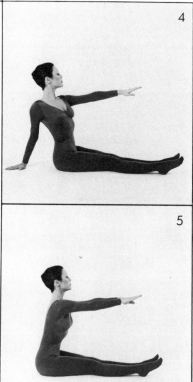

1) Sit on your right side, knees bent, feet together. Place your right hand, fingers spread, at a comfortable distance from your hips. Place your left thumb on your left shoulder. Raise your elbow slightly, forward. Lift your rib cage and lengthen your neck.

2) <u>Plan to keep your right hand on the floor.</u> Keeping your feet on the floor, raise both knees and settle firmly on the buttocks. <u>Your right arm will now be behind you.</u>

3) Raise your left arm smoothly, lift your rib cage and, at the same time, slide your legs forward until they are straight but not stiff. Do not allow your knees to turn out. Without straining, increase the arch of your back.

4) Keeping your rib cage high, lower your left arm to shoulder level with a slight downward pressure. Flex and point your feet firmly 3 times, relaxing after each effort.

5) Lift your right arm and move it forward to shoulder level, staying forward on the buttocks.

4

6) Place your hands on your knees and, without altering your right-angled position, lift and lower your rib cage 6 times. Feel a strong pull in the legs and hips.

7) Flex your feet, then move your hands forward and place them between your ankles and knees. Holding your position, lift and lower your rib cage 6 times. Feel an increased pull along your legs.

8) Plan to relax your hip muscles. Do not curve your back or lift your shoulders. Move your chest forward gradually until your hands touch your toes. Lift and lower your rib cage 6 times. Relax your feet.

9) Lift both arms to shoulder level, then move your right arm behind your hips, placing your right hand on the floor. Stretch forward with the left arm. Lift and lower your rib cage 6 times.

10) Lift and bend your knees and move them to the front. Slide your left arm behind your back. Relax.

Do this sequence 2 times on each side.

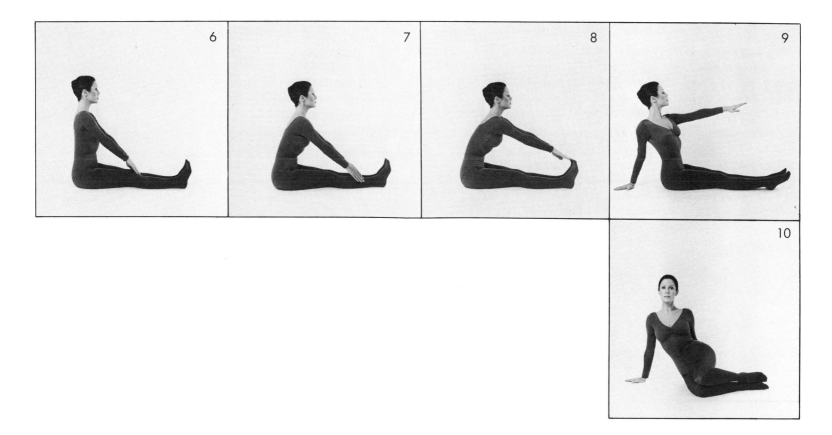

1) On your hands and knees, with hands forward and fingers spread, separate your legs slightly and relax your feet; don't let your toes curl under. Without lifting your chin or straining, hold your head high. Adjust your position so you can support yourself in comfort without overarching.
Shoulders still and arms steady, slowly lift and lower your head 3 times. Relax. Holding your head high, slowly turn it from side to side.

2) With your toes on the floor, slide your left leg back until it is perfectly straight and not turned in or out. Without allowing your hips to move, increase the length of your leg. Hold still as you lift your head and rib cage slightly. <u>Inhale and exhale deeply.</u> Slowly contract your abdomen fully, then relax, 3 times.

3) Press back firmly at the back of your left knee. <u>Feel a strong contraction in the left buttock muscle.</u> This will cause your leg to lift slightly. With head and chest high and your arms and leg perfectly straight, allow your back to arch as you lift your leg as high as possible.

4) Bend your left leg, keeping it high. <u>Feel a strong pull along the front of the thigh.</u>

5) Allowing your spine to curve, lower your left leg and move your knee toward your chest.

6) Move your hands forward the length of one hand. With feet relaxed and arms straight, slowly shift your hips back and lower them to the heels, modifying the position of your hands if necessary. <u>Feel a strong stretching sensation along the back, near the armpits, and along the upper arms.</u> Lower your head and relax.

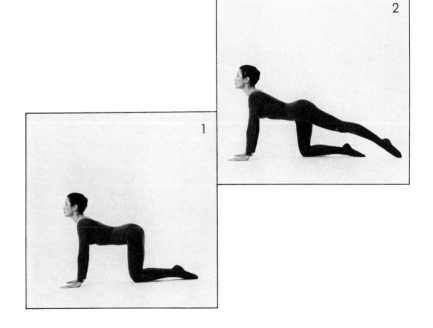

120

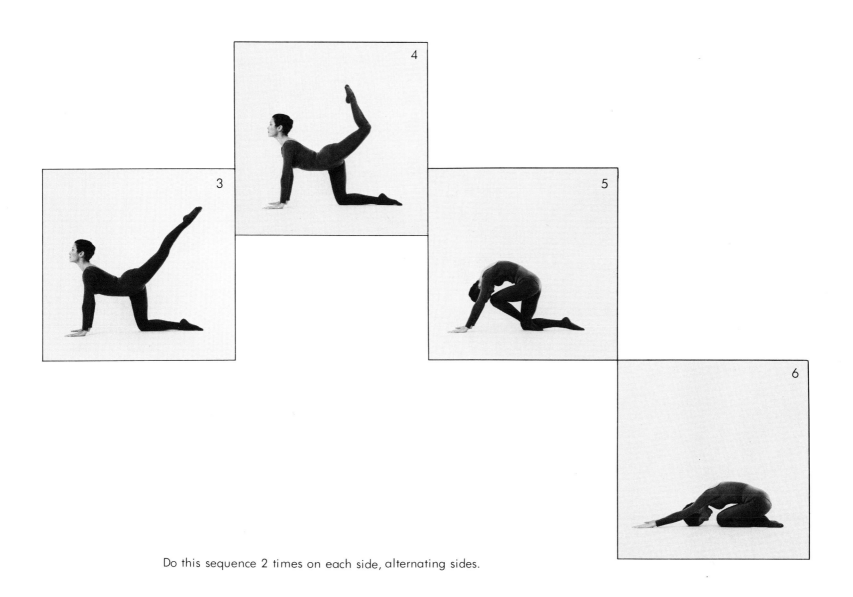

5

Do this sequence 2 times on each side, alternating sides.

5) <u>Plan to keep your left arm straight.</u> Place your left hand at the center of the distance between your right hand and right knee. Straighten your left leg, keeping it slightly behind your hips. <u>Feel a strong pull in the hip, thigh, and groin, and a strong contraction in the buttock.</u>

4) Move your left leg behind you, the left knee touching the right foot, and lift your rib cage high. Relax.

3) Allow your spine to curve as you coax your left knee toward your right shoulder, alternately advancing and releasing it 3 times.

2) Keep your body still as you lift your left leg, placing it behind you so that the left knee touches the right foot. Relax your leg. Lean forward and lift your rib cage. <u>Feel your thigh and lower abdomen tightening.</u>

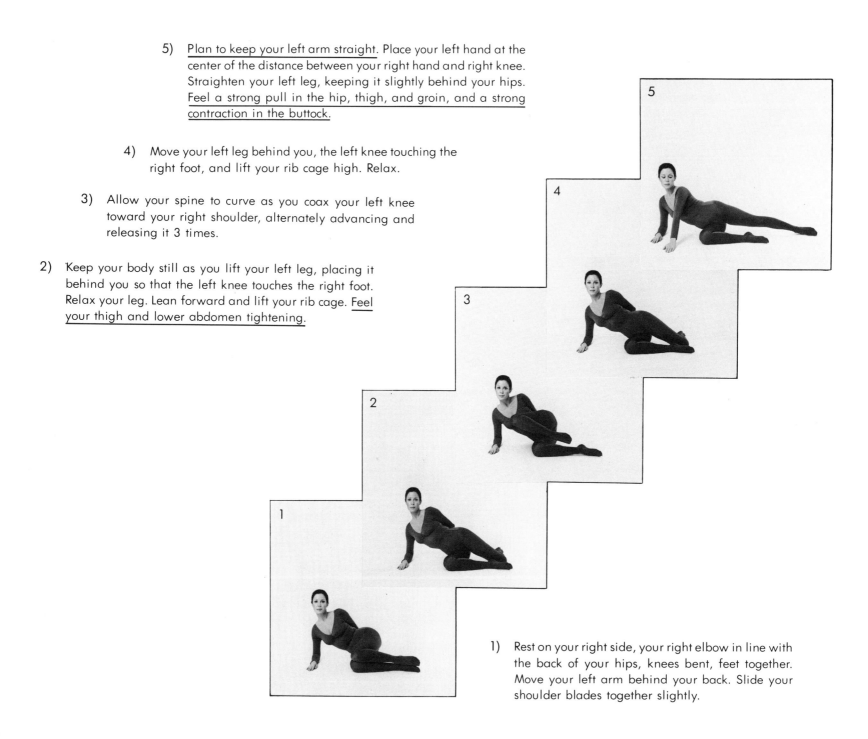

1) Rest on your right side, your right elbow in line with the back of your hips, knees bent, feet together. Move your left arm behind your back. Slide your shoulder blades together slightly.

6) With torso held high, coax your left knee toward your left elbow, alternately advancing and releasing it 3 times. Feel a strong pull in the hip and lower back.

7) Lift your torso and stretch your left leg, pressing firmly back at the knee. Feel a strong contraction in the buttock.

8) Lift and bend your left leg, bringing your knees together. Relax. Lower your head. Inhale, exhale, then contract your abdomen for a slow count of 3. Hold the contraction for a count of 3. Relax and rest for a count of 3. Repeat this part of the pattern 3 times, always inhaling and exhaling before, and resting after each abdominal contraction.

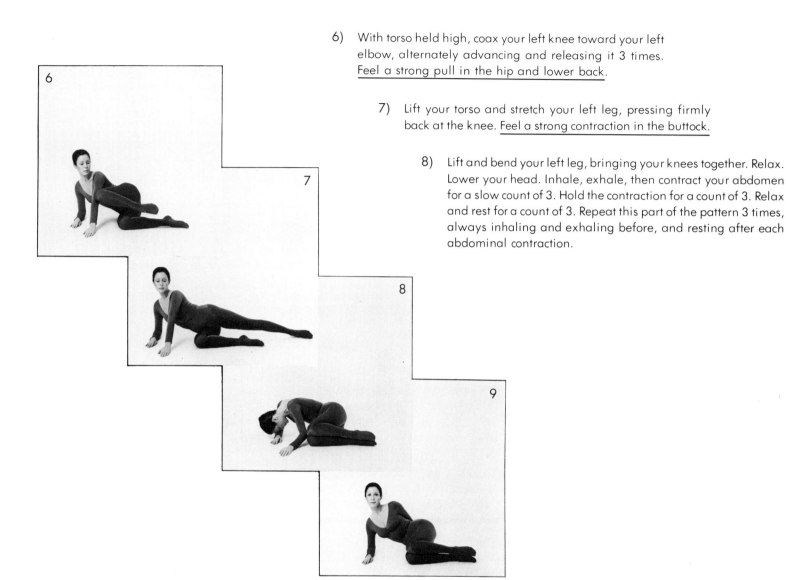

9) Lift your torso, and move back to your starting position. Gently press your shoulder blades together. Relax. Roll your head from the base of your neck 3 times, clockwise and counterclockwise.

Do this sequence 2 times on each side.

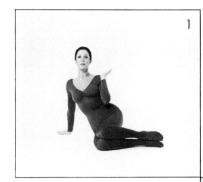

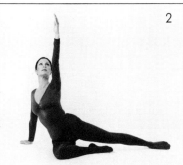

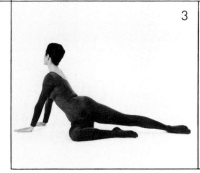

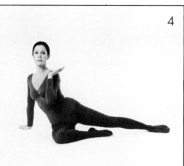

1) Sit on your right side, knees bent, feet together. Place your right hand, with fingers spread, behind your right hip. Place your left thumb on your left shoulder.

2) Slowly move your left arm upward, your left leg to the side, slightly behind your hips. Stretch slowly to full capacity. Feel the stretch in the buttock, thigh, and torso, and the shoulder, arm, and hand. If the effect is not maximal, slide your leg farther back and press the knee back more firmly. Look up at your hand. Relax in position.

3) Plan for the rotation of your torso. Move your right shoulder back, allowing your chest to follow. Lower your left arm and move your left hand toward your right hand. Lift your rib cage. Feel the twisting of muscles in the torso and a strong pull in the hip, buttock, and inner thigh.

4) Place your left thumb on your left shoulder. With rib cage high, rotate your torso back to its original position.

124

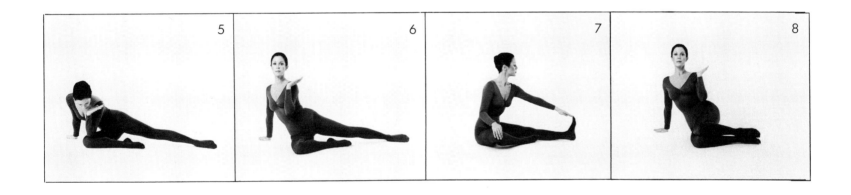

7

5 5) Yielding in the spine, slowly lower your torso until your left elbow touches your right knee. <u>Feel an increased pull at the inner surface of the upper thigh, and a strong pull along your back and hips.</u> Relax in position.

6) Keeping your left thumb against your shoulder, press firmly down in your right palm as you lift your torso. Slide your shoulder blades together slightly and lengthen the back of your neck. Lean slightly forward.

7) Place your right hand on your right knee. As you lower your weight toward your left hip to arrive in a seated position, keep your back straight and move forward on your buttocks. Flex your left foot and do not let your knee turn out. Stretch your left hand as close to your toes as possible, but avoid rounding your back. <u>Feel a strong pull in your hips and leg.</u> Relax.
With your left hand on either your left foot or ankle, alternately bend and straighten your left elbow, moving it in slow up-and-down motion toward and away from your left knee, 6 times. Relax.

8) Resume your starting position.
Do this sequence 3 times on each side.

1) Rest on your back, legs slightly separated, feet relaxed. Place arms at your sides, palms down. Do not lift your chin.

2) Move your shoulder blades together slightly. Palms up, slowly raise your arms, then lower them to the floor beyond your head. Arch your feet. Relax.

3) Bending your knees, place your feet, still slightly separated, firmly on the floor, fairly close to your buttocks. Turn feet out slightly.

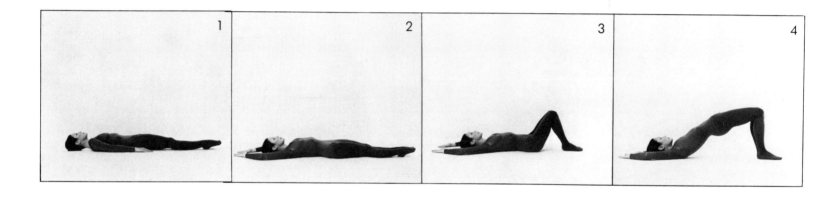

4) Pressing down on your feet, slowly raise your hips. Keep abdomen, neck, and face relaxed. Inhale; exhale; contract your abdomen gradually. Feel your abdomen flattening and firming. Relax. Pressing into your feet, lift your hips a little higher. Inhale; exhale; contract your abdomen gradually. Relax. Slowly lower your hips to the floor.

Repeat the hip lift once in each of the following variations:
1) feet slightly separated and parallel.
2) feet slightly separated and turned in.
Feel different sensations in the legs, hips, and buttocks in different foot positions.

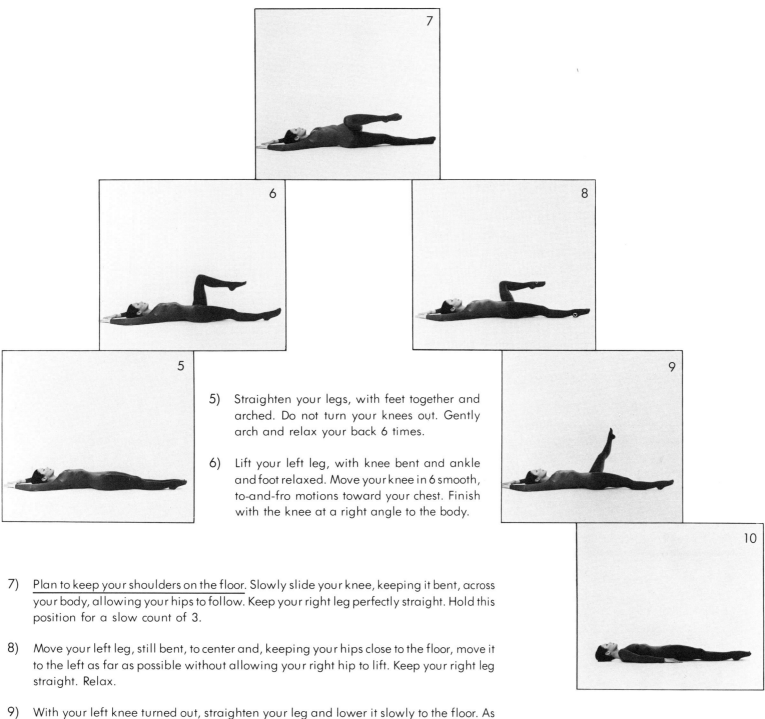

8

5) Straighten your legs, with feet together and arched. Do not turn your knees out. Gently arch and relax your back 6 times.

6) Lift your left leg, with knee bent and ankle and foot relaxed. Move your knee in 6 smooth, to-and-fro motions toward your chest. Finish with the knee at a right angle to the body.

7) <u>Plan to keep your shoulders on the floor.</u> Slowly slide your knee, keeping it bent, across your body, allowing your hips to follow. Keep your right leg perfectly straight. Hold this position for a slow count of 3.

8) Move your left leg, still bent, to center and, keeping your hips close to the floor, move it to the left as far as possible without allowing your right hip to lift. Keep your right leg straight. Relax.

9) With your left knee turned out, straighten your leg and lower it slowly to the floor. As the leg is lowered, <u>feel strong contractions in the abdomen and buttocks.</u>

10) Relax. Return to the starting position.

Do this sequence 1 time on each side.

127

1) Rest on your back, feet together and arched, with arms along your sides, palms down.

2) Bend your knees. Place your feet, slightly turned out and separated, fairly close to the buttocks. Press your shoulders down and relax your arms, neck, and face.

3) Press down firmly on your feet and hands as you raise your hips from the floor. Relax your neck.

4) Place your right foot on top of your left knee. Test for balance; if necessary, adjust the position of your left leg.

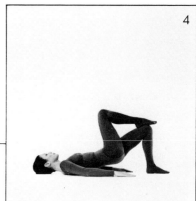

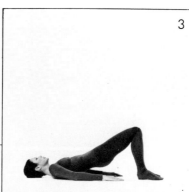

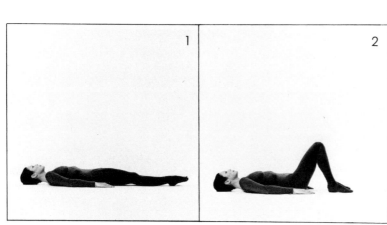

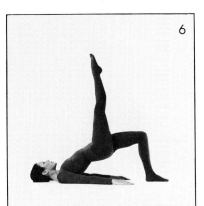

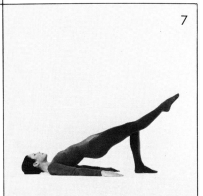

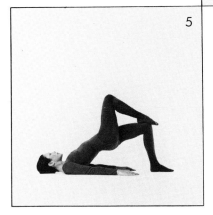

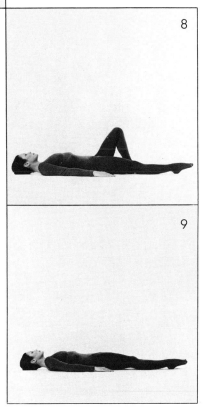

5) Press your right foot firmly down on your left knee and allow your body to arch and lift. Your weight will have shifted toward the shoulders. Do not lift your body too high. Your left leg will carry your weight, contracting strongly in the back of the thigh and calf.

6) Press down on your left foot again and stretch your right leg upward. Your torso will lift slightly. Feel a tightening of muscles in your torso, upper back, and legs. Do not hold this position.

7) Stretch your right leg as you lower it. Stop when your leg is on a level with the left knee. Feel a pull near the groin and lower abdomen.

8) Stretch for a maximum length as you lower your leg and hips to the floor. Relax and rest.

9) Straighten your left leg and allow your knees to roll out. Relax your arms. Slowly roll your head from side to side 6 times.

Do this sequence 3 times on each side.

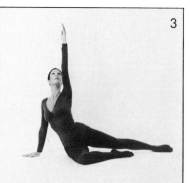

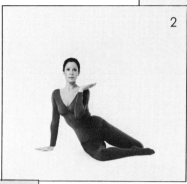

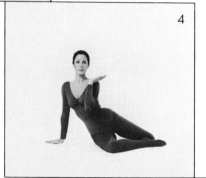

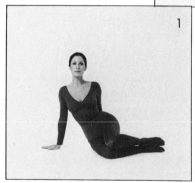

1) Sit on your right side, knees bent, feet together, your right hand at a comfortable distance from the hips. Turn the well of your elbow forward. Feel a tightening at the inner surface of your upper arm. Brace your weight on your right hand and lean slightly forward. Lifting your rib cage, place your left arm behind your back.

2) Do not let your torso sag toward your right hand. Place your left thumb on your left shoulder. Lift your left leg, with knee bent, and place it behind you so that the left knee touches the right foot. Relax your leg; lift your rib cage. Feel a strong pull in the left thigh, buttock, and hip.

3) Slowly move your left arm upward, and look at your hand as you straighten your left leg slightly behind your hip. Lean forward slightly and stretch fully. Feel a powerful pull along your leg and hip, and a strong contraction in the buttock.

5) Bend your right arm, then stretch with an easy sweep toward the right, stretching your left arm and leg fully. Strive for a total stretch. Feel a strong pull along your body and a wrapping sensation in the inner thigh. Hold for a slow count of 3. Relax in position for a slow count of 3.

4) Bend your left leg again, its knee touching your right foot. Lower your left arm, placing your thumb on your left shoulder. Lift your rib cage, and lean forward slightly.

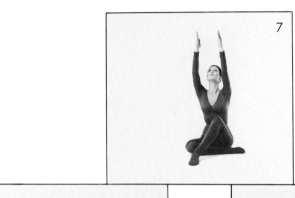

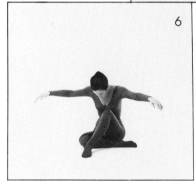

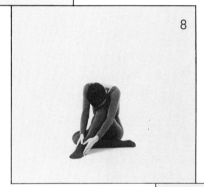

8) In a melting manner, roll your torso slowly forward, lowering your arms and head. Place both hands on your left foot. Relax for a count of 6.

9) Slowly lift your head and torso, and place your right hand on the floor in line with your hips. Move your left leg back, with its knee touching your right foot. Move your left arm behind your back. Arch and stretch your torso.

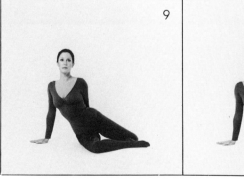

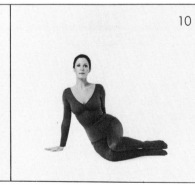

6) Swing your torso upward and your left knee forward to arrive in a seated position, with your left foot turned out in front of your right knee and with both arms extended at shoulder level. Allow your back to curve and lower your head. Settle firmly on your buttocks. Relax in position.

7) Slowly raise your rib cage as you lift your arms above your head and straighten your back. Stretch up from the center of your armpits. Feel a strong pull in the upper back and chest.

10) Move your left leg forward, as in your starting position. Rotate your head from the base of your neck 3 times in both directions.

   Do this sequence 3 times on each side.

Maintenance Program

Even if you are in excellent condition, you are continually exposed to forces that cause tension and threaten to undermine your vitality. To replenish your stores of nervous and muscular energy, continue to practice for a few minutes each day. Alternate between the following programs and the program in the Book of Stretches. You may find it helpful to write each program down on a separate file card and to use markers for the pages you will want to find.

program

1

1) Practice for 3 days:

All Articulations, once each.

Posture Toning 4 to 6, all repeats.

Basic Stretches 1 to 4, twice each.

2) Practice for 3 days:

All Articulations, once each.

Posture Toning 7 to 9, all repeats.

Basic Stretches 5 to 8 twice each.

3) Practice for 3 days:

All Articulations, all repeats.

Posture Toning 8 and 9, all repeats.

Basic Stretches 9 and 10, twice each.

Use the same formula for Dynamic Stretches.

program

2

1) Practice for 3 days:

All Articulations, once each.

Posture Toning 8 and 9, all repeats.

Patterned Stretches 1 to 3, twice each.

2) Practice for 3 days:

All Articulations, once each.

Posture Toning 8 and 9, all repeats.

Patterned Stretches 4 to 6, twice each.

3)   Practice for 3 days:

All Articulations, all repeats.

Posture Toning 8, all repeats.

Patterned Stretches 7 to 10, twice each.

program

3

Practice for 3 days:

All Articulations, once each.

Posture Toning 8, all repeats.

Basic Stretch 1, twice.

Dynamic Stretch 1, twice.

Patterned Stretch 1, twice.

Use the same formula until you have completed all Patterned Stretches.

mini program

Articulations, Sets A and F, all repeats.

Posture Toning 9, all repeats.

Reread "Tension Brakes" on page 60.

Your Programs, by helping you to relax, contribute to your serenity, while a reasonable amount of energy output maintains your strength. Continue to practice, to retard the aging process and to preserve your dynamic vitality.

program guide

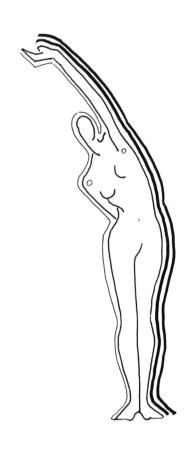